# Parenting Made Complicated

# Parenting Made Complicated

*What Science Really Knows About the*
*Greatest Debates of Early Childhood*

DAVID RETTEW, MD

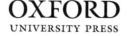

OXFORD
UNIVERSITY PRESS

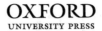

# OXFORD
## UNIVERSITY PRESS

Oxford University Press is a department of the University of Oxford. It furthers
the University's objective of excellence in research, scholarship, and education
by publishing worldwide. Oxford is a registered trade mark of Oxford University
Press in the UK and certain other countries.

Published in the United States of America by Oxford University Press
198 Madison Avenue, New York, NY 10016, United States of America.

Library of Congress Cataloging-in-Publication Data
Names: Rettew, David, author.
Title: Parenting made complicated : what science really knows about the greatest
debates of early childhood / by David Rettew, MD.
Description: New York, NY : Oxford University Press, [2021] |
Includes bibliographical references and index.
Identifiers: LCCN 2020036526 (print) | LCCN 2020036527 (ebook) |
ISBN 9780197550977 (hardback) | ISBN 9780197550991 (epub) |
ISBN 9780197551004 (oso)
Subjects: LCSH: Parenting. | Parent and child. | Child development.
Classification: LCC HQ755.8 .R468 2021 (print) |
LCC HQ755.8 (ebook) | DDC 649/.1—dc23
LC record available at https://lccn.loc.gov/2020036526
LC ebook record available at https://lccn.loc.gov/2020036527

DOI: 10.1093/oso/9780197550977.001.0001

3 5 7 9 8 6 4 2

Printed by Sheridan Books, Inc., United States of America

*This book is dedicated to my mother, Sally, and my father, John, who gave me lots of the love and limits that I needed, although I may not have always appreciated it.*

Also by David Rettew
*Child Temperament: New Thinking About the Boundaries Between Traits and Illness*

# Contents

# Acknowledgments

This book is the product of a very long journey, so there are many people to thank along the way. As described in the first chapter, the idea for the book came 20 years ago from a question about the safety of sleep training that was asked by the mother of one of my patients and whose name I unfortunately have long forgotten. I first brought up the idea for the book soon after that in a supervision session with Dr. Gene Beresin at Massachusetts General Hospital. He very easily could have told me that I had other things on my plate at the time than book writing, but instead his advice was to stop *talking* about the book and get to *writing* it, before someone else does.

I finally did, and I am grateful to people like Dr. Jim Hudziak, Director of Child & Adolescent Psychiatry at the University of Vermont Medical Center, for helping me find time to write while still keeping my day job. I also want to thank Dr. Jess Shatkin, author of *Born to Be Wild*, who offered his expertise in publishing as well as introducing me to some key people, such as literary agent Bonnie Solow who worked with me during the early stages of this process and helped me make the book more accessible to general readers. Two editors, Kittie Moore and Christine Benton, at the book's first home, Guilford Press, also deserve recognition for pushing the book in a direction that it needed to go.

My editor in chief at Oxford University Press, Abby Gross, took a chance in taking me back as an author when this project was suddenly without a publisher. I'm very grateful to her for doing this and hope she is pleased with the outcome of her decision. Thanks also to assistant editor Katherine Pratt, production editor Prabha Karunakaran, and lots of other people I've never had the chance to meet or thank personally who helped this book become real, as well as Holly Watson in publicity relations for her efforts to make as many people as possible aware of this effort.

Of course, big thank-yous also need to be given to my family. My brother Jim designed and supported the book's website. I'm also incredibly thankful for my wife, Valerie, who gave me continued support and inspiration even when I was starting to have my doubts that this project would ever see the inside of a production facility. Finally, I want to thank my three wonderful sons who have made fatherhood such a wonderful experience and have taught me as much if not more than I've taught them.

# PART 1
# GENERAL PRINCIPLES

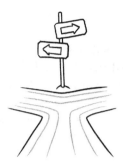

# 1

# It Depends

## Unpacking the Most Boring Answer in Science

All kids need love. All kids need limits.
After that, things can get complicated.

Fortunately for us, we have lots of help when it comes to finding answers to the most debated and vexing questions in parentdom. There's advice on discipline from the overbearing grandfather who swears that "a good spanking" worked for him and should therefore work for everyone, guidance about picky eating from the know-it-all friend whose toddler devoured liver and onions at age two, and tips from the nosy male boss who is just a little too comfortable talking about the health benefits of breastfeeding. And, of course, these days, the modern parent can also look to the seemingly endless quantity of books, articles, blogs, and television shows—all of which seem to arrive at *different* conclusions.

Parental advice from friends and relatives is nothing new, but guidance from total strangers is a relatively recent phenomenon. Dr. Benjamin Spock's 1946 classic book, *Baby and Child Care*, now in its ninth edition,[1] ushered in a wave of parenting guidebooks, despite the somewhat ironic fact that one of the author's central messages was that parents should feel comfortable trusting their *own* instincts. Yet the more investigating you do to find that "correct" answer, the more puzzled you often can become. There is no one more confident about a

Chapter illustrations drawn by Jaq Fagnant

*Parenting Made Complicated.* David C. Rettew, Oxford University Press (2021). © Oxford University Press.
DOI: 10.1093/oso/9780197550977.003.0001

parenting topic than the person who has just finished reading one book on the subject, and no one less confident than the person who has finished two.

Are time-outs effective discipline or abuse? Do children develop better with a stay at home parent or in a daycare? Should I let my toddler play video games? Are kids these days getting too much praise? These are the kinds of questions that so many moms and dads want answered in trying to be the best parents and caretakers that they can. The difficulty isn't finding someone who will give them a definite answer; the difficulty is in finding two people who will give them the *same* answer.

There are a number of reasons why it can be so hard to get a consistent response to what sound like straightforward questions. Some of them have to do with the complexity of human brain and the way that scientific data about parenting is *created*, while others have to do with the way those data are *conveyed*. One of the most important things to realize about most parenting guidance is that it tends to come less in the form of a buffet of options and more like a legal argument a lawyer would make to steer a jury to a particular foregone conclusion. Authors of parenting books and blogs generally stake out a particular thesis on something, like modern parents are too indulgent these days or that screens are destroying developing brains, and then try to get as many people as possible to agree with them. Some carefully selected scientific data are very often *used* to strengthen a particular argument, but that's quite different from an opinion that is necessarily *based* on a careful weighing of the available information. If there is some quality information that argues against an author's central premise, that evidence is most likely going to be ignored rather than incorporated.

All this means that if you want to understand the argument for another perspective, you need to read a *different* book or article and hear about just those studies that support the other view. It's a lot of work, suffering through everyone's best sales pitch and trying to act like some sort of judge while attorneys from opposing sides present their best case. And while this adversarial process may work okay in the courts, it is my view that such a system is less helpful to a parent who is trying in good faith and with an open mind to make important and reasonable decisions about their child. In fact, I'll go a little further and contend that this necessary burden of trying to separate substance from hype in the quest for reliable parenting information results in a lot of us becoming cynical and frustrated with the whole process.

Does it have to be this way? Absolutely not. And, to be fair, there certainly are examples of parenting resources that present information with a minimum of spin, although these tend to be the exceptions to the rule. Why things exist this way isn't clear, but may have something to do with the way people prefer to receive information, or at least the way that most publishers *think* people prefer to receive information. Readers not only want to be educated, but also entertained—and validated. Sure, there is there is a vast scientific literature that bears directly on many of the perennially debated parenting controversies, but that science is complex, indecisive, and sometimes outright contradictory. As a result, one of the most common responses a bona fide child behavior expert is likely to give when asked a tough parenting question, especially one about a particular child, is, "It depends." Such an answer might be true enough, but, oh, is it boring, not to mention unactionable.

"Depends on what?" an eager parent might persist. After all, parents are not looking for guidance about how best to approach the average child from a group of 100 subjects, they are looking for guidance about how to parent *their* child. This is where child temperament, the foundation for what eventually becomes our personality, comes in. Some kids are emotionally fragile while others are resilient. Some crave novelty and adventure while others shy away from it. Some are quite perfectionistic while others couldn't care less about making mistakes. Science often confirms what many parents instinctively know, which is that the conventional one-size-fits-all approach to parenting advice usually falls short— so why do most parenting books continue to treat children as though they are all the same?

This book is designed to be an alternative to the sermons that try to tell you what to think about parenting questions and then push you to apply those same recommendations universally, regardless of other relevant circumstances or what your child is actually like. It's meant not to change the feelings in your gut but rather to enhance the thoughts in your brain. For each parenting dilemma that is presented, my hope is to present to you a summary and synthesis of what science *actually knows* about that particular topic and how solid that level of evidence is at this point. If the overall answer to a particular question is, "It depends," and (spoiler alert) it often is, then we'll look at how that answer may need to be refined or tweaked based on other factors, including the particular temperamental traits of the child and also, sometimes, the parent.

From the outset, it is important to say that I don't believe that scientific evidence should be the only basis by which parenting decisions are made, but maybe it should have a nice seat at the table. The choices we make as parents are based on many things. Often, our parenting policies and practices are not even *choices* at all but rather responses and reactions that follow naturally from our own upbringing, personality, culture, political beliefs, mood, and religion. We remember from our own childhoods what didn't happen but should have, and the hardships we were forced to endure that our own kids hopefully could be spared.

There, of course, is nothing wrong with using these factors in forming our parenting approach. If you believe, for example, that spanking a child is morally wrong, then the degree to which science indicates that spanking "works" in the moment doesn't much matter. If staying home to raise your infant just isn't a financially viable option, then that's the choice that needs to be made, period. The point here isn't that parents should discard intuition, moral codes, and practical realities in their approach to raising children but rather to appreciate that some reliable scientific evidence does actually exist about many of the common parenting debates and is deserving of being heard—especially if it can be distilled and summarized in way that doesn't require a PhD in child development to understand.

## Your Inner Scientist With the Lumpy Oatmeal

In many ways, the pitch here is to encourage parents to act a little more like scientists in two main ways. The first, as has already been mentioned, is to make an effort to try to learn about what is out there with regard to scientific studies in psychology, psychiatry, and child development that relate to many of the practical issues facing parents today. If you have picked up this book, then this likely is already a goal. And if you stay with it, I can confidently tell you that, by the end of this book, you will know more about the science behind some of the most pervasive and debated parenting controversies than the average pediatrician or child psychiatrist.

The second suggestion related to the channeling of your inner scientist, however, requires more than just thoughtful and attentive reading and entails the ability to apply the scientific method to your day to day interactions with children. For those readers who took Psychology 101, this doesn't mean putting your kids in a box to see how often they will press a lever for food. Rather, it involves a transition from a more reactive and dogmatic mode of parenting to a more flexible and inquisitive one. It involves putting the brakes on our most automatic responses as parents to pause and consider our *options*. Then, after we've made a real decision, we observe the consequences of that decision with a flexible mind to see whether or not it made things better. If not, we consider the possibility of choosing a different option in the future.

To make this concept clearer, consider the ubiquitous 3-year-old temper tantrum that erupts over something really stupid. It's 7 o'clock in the morning on a Tuesday. You are rushing to get out the door to work and pretty sure that your daughter knows that. You were hoping she'd be satisfied with a quick breakfast of cereal and milk, but, of course, she insists on having warm oatmeal this morning. Using the raw scientist talents you have already, you bite down on your urge to argue and quickly calculate that the extra 3 minutes it will take to make the oatmeal is probably a wise investment in thwarting what might otherwise be an extended meltdown. You whip up the oatmeal in record time and present it to your daughter with your most encouraging smile.

"There you go sweetie. So yummy!"

She looks at the bowl with a crestfallen look.

"I don't like it," she says. Her shoulders start to slump and her chin falls down to her chest.

"You haven't even tried it," you say, trying to stay positive.

"I don't like it," your daughter repeats. "It's *lumpy*!"

"The oatmeal is fine!" you say, raising your voice. Now you really are late.

"This is just like I make it every other time. You need to eat your breakfast *now*! I don't have time for this nonsense today (except maybe you don't say *nonsense*)!"

Then she starts wailing, and no oatmeal is getting eaten. Now what do you do? For most of us, managing temper tantrums is not easy. Our own emotions start running hot, often fueled by swirling thoughts (my boss is going to be mad, a good parent wouldn't be in the situation, why the **** does my husband never deal with this?) that raise the temperature even higher. Under these circumstances, it is quite understandable that what often happens next is ruled by the emotional part of our brain rather than the rational part. Then we yell, we criticize, and do lots of things other than *think*.

But what if we are able to keep that little scientist on our shoulder a bit longer as the child's tears begin to fall? Maybe then we can continue to hold in our mind the thought that we really have some choices as parents when a toddler begins to get upset. Option no. 1: we can calmly walk away (under the idea that this display is really a push for attention). Option no. 2: we can stoop down and try to coach the daughter in calming down (under the idea that she can't regulate herself in the moment and needs some help). Option no. 3: we can pick up the oatmeal and throw it in the trash (under the idea that we shouldn't reinforce temper tantrums as a way to get what you want). Each of these options has some merit to support it as a strategy, but which one will work best for an individual child at that precise moment depends on a lot of moving parts that may be hard to predict. Picking the best approach requires first a parent being able to keep their head while thinking through the options, then choosing one of those options based on the best evidence at the time and testing it for a while to see what happens, evaluating the result, and finally, having the courage to make adjustments if the initial guess didn't work out.

This, in a nutshell, is what the scientific method is all about. We study the scientific evidence, we make a hypothesis based on that information, we test that hypothesis with our own data, and if necessary, we adjust that hypothesis and start again. Of course, being able to pull this off in the real world of parenting can be a major challenge. We'll never do this perfectly, but that's okay. Just by making a commitment to try to parent based on what we learn, attempt, and observe, we incrementally free ourselves from falling into the same holes over and over again as we move toward an approach that is rational, informed, and, perhaps more than anything, *deliberate*.

## Where This Book Came From

It's hard to underestimate just how much trepidation I have in being viewed as a parenting "expert." I often joke that being a child psychiatrist doesn't render you immune to making all the same mistakes that every other parent does; it just makes you much more acutely *aware* of those mistakes. Over the years, I've attended more than my fair share of parenting-oriented presentations and lectures. I usually leave them feeling pretty impressed with the speaker and his or her ability to raise happy and healthy children. Unfortunately, I also tend to wind up feeling even more deficient regarding my own skills rather than empowered to carry out those strategies myself. Sometimes, it seems as though the best thing I could do to benefit my own children is to figure out how to get the speaker to adopt them.

This book hopefully won't be one of those experiences for you. While many parenting authors trace the motivation for their book to an event that revealed their level of parenting acumen, my seminal event was all about demonstrating my level of parenting ignorance. I was still in training as a child psychiatry fellow after having finished both medical school and a general psychiatry residency program. I was thus closing in on an entire decade of training in my chosen field, which means that I definitely should have learned a thing or two by this point. I was doing some psychotherapy with an 8-year-old boy who, among other things, was not particularly thrilled with having a 2-year-old sister sucking up all of the parental energy. In meeting with the boy's mother, she told me about how hard it was to devote the needed attention to both children, particularly because she always felt so tired on account of the daughter still waking up multiple times per night. She mentioned that she and her husband were thinking of "Ferberizing" their daughter to help her sleep through the night but were confused over the mixed messages they had heard in the media about doing that. She then asked me what I had been taught on the subject and what I thought she should do to help everyone get a better night's rest.

In that moment, I tried to run through the hundreds of lectures and seminars I'd heard on a huge range of topics. I was training at the one of the most respected and prestigious psychiatry programs in the country. Top experts had spoken to us about the genetics of schizophrenia, Freud's theory of psychosexual develop-ment, brain scans, and the pros and cons of various antidepressants, but remark-ably, I couldn't recall a single session about the nuts and bolts of parenting and the common dilemmas parents often face. Was this not an important topic? Was there no published science on these kinds of questions? It suddenly seemed bi-zarre that such a huge gaping hole could exist in my otherwise world-class educa-tion. I told the mother that this was an excellent question and that I would need to do some additional investigation and get back to her. Nearly 20 years later, with that daughter now probably finishing college, I finally have.

## The Muddy Waters of Parenting Science

In the course of my inspired efforts to learn as much as I can about the science of parenting, I've read countless numbers of research studies, reviews of those studies, and supercharged meta-analyses that try to combine data from many re-search studies into one big data set. I've also taken myself out of the academic lit-erature to look at trade books, magazine articles, and blogs that attempt to make sense of this vast science. In the process, I've learned that the wide-ranging and often contradictory views that get expressed are not only due to the particular characteristics of the many messengers out there but also a product of the science itself.

Research on parenting is definitely science, but it's not the kind of science that most people think of when envisioning serious-looking people with dishev-eled white hair in lab coats transferring bubbling liquids from one test tube to another. Many of us might remember as schoolchildren the task of replicating Galileo's famous experiment from the Tower of Pisa in which he demonstrated that two objects dropped at the same time hit the earth at the same moment even if one object is heavier than the other. What made this a popular lesson for kids learning the scientific method wasn't just the fact that you got to drop things from high up and watch them crash to the ground. Rather, teachers liked it be-cause it *worked* and, specifically, because it was *replicable*. With one force being evaluated, namely gravity, it was possible to get the same answer every time from place to place, experimenter to experimenter.

Medical and behavioral science, however, work very differently. The subjects now are people or animals rather than objects, and there are a huge number of often hard to measure factors that play a role in determining why things happen the way they do. Even a seemingly straightforward experiment like testing whether or not a new medication works is likely to get a little messy. Suppose, for example, you are a medical scientist trying to test a new antibiotic for children with ear infections. You get 100 children with documented ear infections who agree to be part of your experiment. Then, after an initial visit to confirm the infection, half of the people get a prescription for the new antibiotic and half get a sugar pill or placebo. After a week, all the patients come back, and the main variable of interest is whether or not their ear infection has resolved.

If things worked like the Galileo experiment, everything would be simple: all of the people who got the new antibiotic would get better and all of the children who got placebo would not. Then the scientist could very confidently state that the drug was effective in treating ear infections. But we all know that such a scenario almost never happens. Due to variables like the strength of the infection, the type of bacteria or virus, and how strong an individual child's immune system is, there are going to be people who get the drug who don't clear the infection, and kids who get placebo who do. There's also likely to be children who get *a little* better, but not all the way. Now what? If 60% of the kids who got the antibiotic improved compared to 40% of kids in the placebo, is that good enough evidence that the antibiotic "works," or could those numbers just have occurred from chance?

Things get even more challenging in naturalistic studies that don't involve the gold standard of subjects being randomized to one situation versus another, which is most of the parenting research. Why most studies exist without randomization is not hard to understand. Suppose, for example, a parenting researcher wanted to look at the impact of spanking on long-term behavior (a topic of one of the chapters in this book). In designing the definitive study, the researcher would want to recruit a large number of families from a variety of ethnic and socioeconomic backgrounds. She then would want to randomize the subjects into two groups with one that would be carefully trained to use spanking as a disciplinary technique under very specific circumstances, while the other group would agree never to use spanking for any situation for the next, say, 8 years. This randomization procedure would be very important scientifically because it would maximize our confidence that any behavioral differences found between kids in the two groups was caused by the spanking or nonspanking rather than something else.

Spanking and the impact of various kinds of disciplinary strategies is a very important issue for parents, and a study like this would really go a long way to answer the long-standing debate about whether corporal punishment is good or harmful to children. Yet this study previously described has yet to be done. Why? Primarily because the vast majority of parents would never let a flip of the coin decide whether or not they are going to use spanking as a punishment for the next several years of a child's life, and the ones who would allow themselves to be randomized this way probably don't represent the population of parents as a whole.

To circumvent these problems, researchers are compelled to forgo the randomization and simply survey some families who spank their children and some who don't and apply questionnaires to measure how well-behaved their children are. This could provide some useful information, but it is going to be very challenging to eliminate the possibility that factors other than the spanking are responsible for any differences in child behavior. Maybe child aggression is really due to genetics with more aggressive parents passing down those "aggressive" genes to their kids. Since those aggressive parents also spank more, then what looks like a parental effect of spanking on a child's level of aggression may actually be masking a true genetic effect. Or suppose we find that spanked children are more well-behaved than kids who are never spanked, but families who spank also tend to be more structured and set better limits than nonspanking families. If that good behavior is really a function of that increased structure and limits and the study doesn't do a good job of measuring and accounting for those other variables, then it might mistakenly look like the spanking is what really matters when it isn't.

Since it is nearly impossible to account for all the potentially important moving parts that can cloud up the ability to make a "beyond a reasonable doubt" conclusion, all studies contain those proverbial *flaws* that can be used by critics to discredit the study. And here is where the human element creeps back into science. With so much wiggle room in the data, a parenting expert's bias can start to take over, consciously or not. When that happens, we can start doing things like being more vigilant of the flaws in studies that don't conform to our current beliefs while giving similarly flawed studies that reinforce our views a pass. We can do a little cherry-picking with regard to what studies we choose to highlight in support of one position or another. And once a person has staked a particular position on an issue *publicly* in a book or a blog, it's even harder to change your mind lest you be seen as traitorous to your followers or, even worse, wishy washy. If you spent some time in the world of parenting advice, you know that the books and articles that are published come from authors of diverse backgrounds: reporters, nutritionists, attorneys, and, for some reason, a disproportionate number of economists—most of whom are also experienced parents. A lot of parenting books aren't written by people with training in child development or behavior. To be fair, many of these publications offer solid advice and often summarize the scientific evidence quite well. But at the risk of sounding like a snob, there are some advantages to having spent years both as a mental health clinician who has worked with thousands of children and families on behavioral challenges and as a researcher who has actually contributed to the behavioral science database. Working clinically as a child psychiatrist has shown me just how wildly diverse kids and their environments can be and why we can't possibly think that some decree from on high about what all parents should do is going to provide universal benefit. As an academic and a researcher, I've learned the way science really works: both its noble qualities that compel us to pay attention and its more shadowy alleyways where bias, politics, and greed can exert more influence than we would like to admit. As the late great Sir George Michael once sang, "I know all the games you play, because I play them too."

## Goals of This Book

It would be incredibly naïve of me to claim, after all this, that I am going to provide you with a truly objective and totally complete view of the science behind many of the most debated topics facing parents today and how that science might be customized to suit individual children. Nevertheless, that's the plan.

I have to confess that writing this book has led me to challenge some of my own preconceptions. As a father of three children, my own natural parenting approach, like everyone else's, is an extension of my own experiences, beliefs, and bits of knowledge picked up on the way. As a scientist, however, we are taught not to hold on to our ideas too firmly, lest we become unable to follow our data to their eventual conclusions. One of my favorite bumper stickers, origin unknown, reads, "Don't believe everything you think." This is not an easy task, and the research that I have read and considered has sometimes been "inconvenient" to how I've handled things in the past.

Personally, when I feel someone pushing me to act or think in a certain way, my own inclination is to go in the opposite direction. If that sounds familiar, I hope that you will find the tone of this book to be collegial rather than preachy—one that appeals to you as an educated consumer rather than a lost sheep. In this spirit, *Parenting Made Complicated* will demand from you a bit more than you may be accustomed. You'll need to hang in there for longer than a sound bite. Most of the parenting issues covered in the book are controversial for a reason. It takes time to understand the scientific evidence and real effort to apply it to an individual child. This is not a reference book in which a quick answer to a question can be found on page *x*, although each chapter can be read on its own for readers interested mainly on a smaller number of topics. While most chapters do contain a boxed summary of what the science says about a particular parenting debate and how that overall conclusion might need to be altered based on a child's particular traits or other factors, it is likely that many readers will be impressed with how much we still *don't* know about important subjects and how conflicting the science still is in areas. For some parents, this might feel liberating: a license to move forward as one was inclined to do already. For others, it will be unsettling and perhaps a motivation not to move too far to the extreme on either side. Regardless, most readers willing to dive in here will encounter a great deal of information that you probably never knew existed.

*Parenting Made Complicated* focuses on long-standing debates in parenting that are related to behavior. There are plenty of other parenting controversies out there about birthing or diapers or introducing solid food that are well covered elsewhere and outside my scope of knowledge. Some other topics like the supposed link between vaccines and autism are also left out, because, frankly, there just isn't that much controversy left when it comes to the known science. The chapters also center on debates that arise for younger children up to around age 5, although certainly some of these topics are of concern for parents of older children too.

The book is divided into three main sections. The first deals with more general and overarching concepts. Since one of the main points of this book is that the optimal parenting strategy for a particular child may depend on their (and your) temperament or personality, chapter 2 provides an overview of what temperament is, how it could be measured in children and parents, and why it matters. Chapter 3 then explores what is known about some of the most well-known general approaches to parenting, such as *attachment* or *free-range* parenting, and how these more popular terms fit in with the way scientists have traditionally categorized parenting approaches.

From there, we dive into more specific parenting debates and dilemmas that have been with us for decades and continue to inspire impassioned opinions and discourse. The second section explores controversies that are especially relevant to infants and toddlers. These include the perennial "pick them up versus let them cry" question about sleep training methods, a look at the evidence that breastfeeding can improve a child's cognitive and behavioral development, the vexing choice for many parents about staying home to care for young children versus using daycare or other childcare options, and an exploration into how young children form their identity around gender and how much control parents have in this process. On a related point regarding pronoun use in this book, I often will alternate the pronoun *he* and *she* when describing children in general. This is not meant to imply that the text only refers to one gender but rather is done for conciseness and to avoid more tiresome terms like *he/she*.

The next four chapters focus on topics that tend to be especially related to toddlers and preschoolers. These include approaches to children who are picky eaters, what is known about the effects of parental divorce on children, media usage in young children and how solid the evidence is about its links with behavioral problems like aggression and hyperactivity, and some investigation about the optimal amount and type of praise that children receive. Finally, the last chapter takes a practical look at strategies that could be used by a family to operationalize some of this new knowledge into actual behavioral change. Notice that I use the word *family* rather than *parent*. This is intentional, as the chances of turning the insights you will gain from this book into actual changes that can benefit the development of your child are considerably higher if the other people helping to raise your child (should there be any) also read the book and are part of the process to figure out what, if anything, should be done with this information. This last chapter will help you organize your thoughts and insights into action that adjusts how you may already be parenting your child or how you may be planning to parent your child in the future.

Dispersed within most of the chapters will be boxed clinical vignettes that will help make the science more relevant and illustrate how parents of different children under different circumstances might arrive at diverse conclusions when confronting the same parenting challenge. These cases do not refer to specific individuals or families but do reflect a conglomeration of real-world situations and choices that parents whom I have had the privilege to work with over the years have made. There are also a large number of references that can be identified by their superscript numbers to help reassure you that I am not just making all this stuff up. For those interested in looking at original sources, these references can be found at the back of the book so as not to disrupt the flow of reading.

I suppose that at some point in the chapter I should also mention that the information contained in this book should not be construed as official medical advice for your specific child. In writing this sentence, I am certainly aware that neither I as the writer nor you as the reader are probably here for purely entertainment purposes. Nevertheless, the message is worth stating as there is no substitute for working with a real live professional who understands the individual circumstances of your child and family.

I expect that this book will hardly represent the final word on these important and highly debated topics. Some people are likely to get a little upset about what is written here and will likely criticize various chapters for giving this study too much weight, another too little, or missing some important evidence altogether. In some cases, their feedback will be quite legitimate. All this is okay and part of what makes the progression of science great—when it works well.

## All Parents Should Do This

Finally, a word about the process of how this book came into being. In trying to find a publisher, I ran, of course, into a number of roadblocks and rejections as nearly all authors do. Some of them were inevitably directed at me as the author, but in full disclosure, most of them were directed at *you*, the reader. I was told that the parenting public basically just wants to be told what to do and that readers can't handle more than one major parenting controversy at a time in a single book. Essentially, I heard that parents are just too overwhelmed or too lazy to read something like this.

I don't believe this and am hoping you and my enthusiastic publisher will prove them wrong. Help me demonstrate that a parent can do better by being given options rather than recipes. Help me show the media and publishing world that a moderate stance on an issue can be a sign of strength, not weakness. And in the process, help yourself to becoming as fully informed as you possibly can regarding decisions that you will have to make anyway, one way or another. Parenting is very hard work, and providing love and limits can indeed go quite a long way to help a child meet her full potential. But for the parent eager to learn more about the important and fascinating world of parenting research and how that research can be harnessed to the benefit of your individual child or children, I invite you to read on.

# 2

# Child Temperament 101

## A Primer on Personality Differences in Children

If one of the main drivers of an "it depends" approach to parenting relates to the temperament of your child (and yourself), it makes sense to take some time to explain a bit more about what exactly temperament is. This chapter will offer a short overview on the subject and then give you some tools to be able to rate the temperament of your child, yourself, and really anyone else you know. Those ratings will come in handy later when specific parenting controversies are reviewed relative to kids who vary according to their temperamental predispositions.

One of the first things I had to do as a child psychiatrist in training was to observe typically developing children—the quite reasonable argument being that one needs to have a good grasp about the range of "normal" child behavior before being in a solid position to make psychiatric diagnoses. On a warm summer Tuesday morning in the middle of Boston, our fellowship class of eight were released from our arduous responsibilities at the hospital so that we could watch and interact with kids in their natural environment. These brief excursions were essentially the lab component of our seminar in child development.

The first stop, under the tutelage of our able instructor Paula Rauch, was a public playground in one of the leafier neighborhoods not far from Boston University. "Tell me what you all observe," she instructed us. This invitation at first seemed far too vague, yet just in a matter of minutes some of the rudimentary properties that separated the behavior of some children from others, and the ways parents responded to them, unfolded before our eyes.

Chapter illustrations drawn by Jaq Fagnant

*Parenting Made Complicated.* David C. Rettew, Oxford University Press (2021). © Oxford University Press.
DOI: 10.1093/oso/9780197550977.003.0002

The children were enjoying the colorful playground equipment of swings, tunnels, slides, and a multilayered climbing apparatus, while the parents (mostly moms) hovered nearby at various levels of engagement. The main objective of many of the moms was clearly to prevent their kids from becoming careless and getting hurt. Their frequent admonishments of "That's too high to jump from there!" or "Don't go down head first!" echoed through the trees. Others, by contrast, seemed to be trying to embolden their kids toward taking *greater* risk. One mother urged her daughter to go even higher on the swing, while another provided an encouraging nod to a boy who looked warily at the entrance to a long tunnel. Unfortunately, we didn't get much of a show that first morning, as the sight of nine professionally dressed and childless adults standing around a playground and pointing soon caught the skeptical eye of many parents, who then decided it might be a good idea to go home for a snack.

We then were herded into a van en route to a nearby childcare center where our professor had once taken her own kids. The center was composed of a number of age-based classrooms from infancy all the way through to prekindergarten. Going from class to class, we were able to walk through time as we paid attention to things like language development, motor skills, social behavior, and the complexity of the artwork on the walls.

Yet amidst all the amazing progressions we saw in these areas, some of the original behavioral differences we had so briefly observed on the playground seemed to persist, regardless of age. Within each classroom there were some children who eagerly approached us with curiosity and others who seemed uncomfortable and hesitant. There were some children who moved loudly across the room while others quietly remained in place. There were a few names we heard over and over again in the course of being given "reminders" about their behavior and some who seemed to require almost no adult intervention at all.

Being a new father myself to a then 6-month-old son, I was only too happy to impart my *considerable* wisdom and experience to my classmates, particularly those who were not parents themselves. In the preschool room, as a couple of my fellow fellows stood nervously in the midst of the exuberant chaos, I gave them my most technical advice for winning over the young crowd.

"Sit down!" I told them.

For many of the kids, that literally was all it took before one child would shove a book in your hand while another one climbed on your head. A few, however, needed much more encouragement to engage due to being nervous, preoccupied, or just simply not that interested. After another 30 minutes or so, we departed generally feeling both inspired and exhausted—ready to take a nap of our own.

## What Is Child Temperament?

In the end, it was these basic differences in behavior that captured my interest the most. Over tea at our supervisor's home, we discussed these basic patterns of behaviors as reflective of a child's *temperament*. While academics continue to debate its precise definition, temperament could be practically described as the typical manner to which people approach and react to the world around them. Some folks boldly go where no one has gone before, while others are quite content to stay right where they are, thank you very much. Some people are quickly brought to tears, others to smile, while others require extreme provocation to get any kind of emotional reaction at all. In many ways, temperament can be viewed as the building blocks of one's personality—those early fundamental traits that become further developed and sculpted by the forces of one's environment, experiences, genetics, and time itself. For some kids, these other influences have the effect of strengthening their temperamentally based traits while in other cases these forces push a child's behavior in a different direction.

## Temperament Versus Personality

Throughout these chapters, the terms *temperament* and *personality* will be used interchangeably. They probably shouldn't be as the two terms mean somewhat different things. While both personality and temperament refer to core traits whose levels vary from one person to the next, the label *temperament* is often applied to children while personality isn't thought to fully arrive on the scene until adolescence. The idea here is that the ingredients that form the soup of a personality trait are more complex, including things like more advanced cognitive skills, cultural influences, and accumulating life experiences. Even though the name of a temperament and personality trait might be exactly the same, like extraversion, the temperament version of it that might be observed in a 2-year-old is a bit more, well, *basic*.

Experts, however, still argue over the boundaries between temperament and personality, and it is certainly fair to say that any distinctions between the two domains is at least somewhat arbitrary. For that reason, and for sake of simplicity, we'll leave the academic debates on this subject to the scientific conferences and treat the two constructs as generally the same.

## Negative Emotionality, Extraversion, and Effortful Control

Temperament is usually thought to consist of a small number of broad traits or dimensions that can be broken down into more specific components (or facets).

Given how long little kids have been on this planet, let alone bewildered parents wondering what the heck is going on with these little kids, one might well expect that the whole classification system for child temperament has been pretty well worked out by now. Unfortunately, that is far from reality, and many basic questions regarding the core dimensions of temperament have yet to be fully answered. Those of you who took basic Human Development or Psychology 101 in college may be surprised to hear this because, in many of those classes, it seemed like the world of temperament was so nicely wrapped up decades ago with the research of Chess and Thomas. For those of you who missed it, Stella Chess and Alexander Thomas were two child psychiatrists in New York who in the 1960s and 1970s began publishing work on the well-known New York Longitudinal Study, which closely followed a group of individuals from infancy into adulthood.[1,2] While temperament was certainly not a new concept at the time, Chess and Thomas, along with some others, are credited for really putting it back on the radar screen, particularly for people working clinically with children. Through their observations and some basic statistical methods performed by Herbert Birch, they proposed that children were innately predisposed to have different levels of nine basic temperament traits:

1. Activity level
2. Rhythmicity (i.e., how regular and predictable they are with regard to things like sleeping, eating, and pooping)
3. How much they approach or withdraw from novelty
4. Adaptability to new situations or caregiver demands
5. How intense a stimulus needs to be to trigger a behavioral response
6. The behavioral and emotional intensity of that response once triggered
7. Overall positive versus negative mood
8. Distractibility
9. General attention span and ability to persist on an activity

The idea of a child being born with a predisposition toward particular traits is almost in the no-brainer category today, but back then the ideas were met with scorn and skepticism. At the time, two of the biggest schools of thought with regard to child behavior were psychoanalysis, which postulated that personality traits come from the channeling of unconscious sexual and aggressive drives, and behaviorism, which hypothesizes that children are born a "blank slate," acquiring traits exclusively through learning principles. While these two perspectives were often fiercely at odds with each other, neither of them, at least in their more extreme forms, left much room for the idea of behavioral tendencies that were present from the get-go due to one's genes. Nevertheless, Chess and Thomas endured the criticisms and their work inspired new generations of researchers eager to advance the understanding of child temperament.

And advance they did. In the process, new scholars found that the Chess and Thomas dimensions were a major step forward in the world of temperament research but, as is common with science, needed some refinements. One of those scientists was a psychologist named Mary Rothbart, who worked at the University of Oregon. She and her colleagues conducted a large number of studies with children and adults of all ages, and the result has been the development of one of the most widely used temperament frameworks in the world today.[3,4]

In this system, temperament is thought to consist of three major or primary dimensions, with each one being broken down to more specific traits that are loosely related to each other. The exact composition of these traits under this system is thought to vary slightly depending on the developmental stage (infancy, early childhood, etc.), but in general the structure is fairly consistent across the life span.

### Negative Emotionality

Under this framework, one of the major dimensions is called *negative emotionality* or negative affectivity. This term may sound technical, but an easier way to think of it is how prone a young child is to feeling *stressed*. Going further, negative emotionality refers to the tendency of someone to experience negative emotions such as fear, sadness, and frustration. Infants, toddlers, and preschoolers who score higher in negative emotionality tend to become upset more easily, and, when they do, it can be more difficult to bring them back to baseline. These kids can be reticent and nervous when exposed to new people and new situations, and they can be more easily thrown off course by frustration or anxiety when engaging in challenging tasks. The broad trait of negative emotionality can be broken down to more specific components that include predispositions specifically to anger, fear, sadness, and feeling uncomfortable, as well as being more difficult to soothe. To a toddler who is low in negative emotionality, going for his first haircut may be no big deal (thanks for the lollipop). For the toddler high in negative emotionality, that same haircut can feel like a living nightmare for everyone involved.

### Extraversion

A second major dimension is extraversion, which in more technical circles has also been dubbed *surgency*. In some ways, this dimension is the opposite of negative emotionality and describes children who easily experience positive emotions such as joy and excitement. This dimension also reflects some social characteristics such as being more gregarious and comfortable around people. Young children high in the extraversion dimension like more stimulating activities. As infants, they are more likely to be the ones that squeal with delight when somebody tosses them up into the air and more likely to bolt across the lawn to say hi to the neighbor's dog when Mom looks away for 3 seconds. These kids might often be described as energetic, animated, and adventurous. The subcategories of extraversion/surgency include activity level, enjoyment of high-stimulation activities, joyfulness, lack of shyness, impulsivity, and talkativeness.

### Effortful Control

The third major dimension of temperament, *effortful control*, is a little different. If negative emotionality and extraversion can be conceptualized as emotional-behavioral accelerators that push kids *toward* different kinds of feelings and reactions, effortful control functions more as a *brake*. What is being captured here is a child's ability to regulate her thoughts, feelings, and behavior. A child who is high on effortful control is able to focus on a story being read to her, perhaps because she actually enjoys engaging in slower-paced activities. She may also be a bit better at following the story because she has the ability to hold off other impulses, like running outside to play, when she is told that it's story time. Finally, effortful control in younger children also includes the ability to perceive more subtle aspects and changes of the world around them. When I dropped off my then 4-year-old son (who was hopefully working hard on his effortful control skills) at preschool one day, he remarked how the lines in the parking lot had just been painted. I, of course, was completely oblivious to this change. As children get older, this dimension of effortful control becomes part of what is often referred to as executive functioning skills, such as the ability to plan, delay gratification, self-monitor, and think in an organized manner. These capabilities, as you might expect, are strongly associated with a number of positive outcomes including longer life, higher income, and increased happiness.[5]

### Five Kinds of Kids (At Least)

These three dimensions of temperament—negative emotionality, extraversion/surgency, and effortful control—are thought to be mostly independent of each other. Being high or low on one dimension thus does not predict one's score on another dimension. That said, their interrelations are not random, and studies indicate that higher levels of negative emotionality are weakly related to lower levels of extraversion/surgency, and vice versa.[6] Higher levels of effortful control also have a habit of being somewhat related to lower levels of both negative emotionality and extraversion/surgency. Plenty of parents, however, will know of exceptions to this rule—like the child who very much want to be part of everything going on around him (high extraversion) but then often becomes easily flustered and distressed in the process (high negative emotionality).

So far, we have focused our understanding of child temperamental traits on the level of the individual dimensions themselves. Another equally valid perspective is to broaden our view or "unit of study" and focus not on each temperament dimension itself but rather on an individual's particular profile across all of the major temperament dimensions. For example, one of your children might be low on negative emotionality and high on both extraversion and effortful control.

After spending a lot of time observing children, it becomes evident that certain *constellations* of temperamental traits seem to appear in kids over and over again. (Yes, of course it is true that children are like snowflakes with no two being exactly the same temperamentally, but it is also true that particular combinations of traits exist together more frequently than would be predicted by chance alone.) Perhaps the most famous of these temperament types is the "difficult" child proposed by Chess and Thomas many decades ago. Encompassing about 10% of young children, this term describes kids who can have trouble adapting to new situations, are often sad or irritable, are prone to big emotional outbursts, and often show irregular sleep and eating patterns.[7]

Computers now can do this kind of pattern recognition too, and when you run certain kinds of statistical analyses on large groups of children, what often pops out is the identification of three to six temperament types who tend to have similar levels of traits A, B, and C. These distinct types have been identified for children as young as 18 months of age[8] with early manifestations of these types being evident even earlier.[9] Our research group at the University of Vermont, in collaboration with others, has taken a couple of stabs at these kinds of studies as well, once with a sample of American children who were selected to have relatively high rates of behavioral problems[10] and another with a Flemish sample in Belgium.[11] Unfortunately, the computer doesn't spit out the proper *names* for the different types; that you have to do yourself, and it can be one of the more difficult aspects of the whole project. In both studies, however, we identified a more "average" group that had medium levels of all of the temperament dimensions. People in the past[8] have called this group "unremarkable," but to us that just sounded a bit derogatory (would you want to have an "unremarkable" child?) so we used the term *moderate* instead. Other types we labeled "disengaged" and "steady," although now I'm not sure those were the best choices.

As you can imagine, coming up with a consensus within the academic world for child temperament types is no easier than agreeing over the number and names of the primary dimensions. Despite these challenges, I attempted in my last book to propose the existence of five main temperament types based on the available research.[12] These types, which will be used for discussion in future chapters regarding the big parenting debates, are as follows:

1. *Anxious.* This temperament type is similar to older terms such as "overcontrolled" or "slow to warm up" and describes children who tend to be higher on negative affectivity and lower on extraversion/surgency. Many of them also struggle with lower levels of effortful control. These kids are easily upset, often seem uncomfortable, and can be difficult to soothe. They also don't tend to take to new people and situations without a lot of parental encouragement.

2. *Vigorous.* The vigorous type of child is high in extraversion and low in negative affectivity. Children belonging to this type are active, sometimes fearless, and eagerly approach new situations. They like to be swung up high and enjoy rough-and-tumble play. They may, however, get angry or aggressive if there is an obstacle in the way of what they want. They may also get themselves in trouble through a lack of caution and restraint. Other researchers have used terms like *resilient* or *confident.*

3. *Agitated.* Children with the agitated profile have a somewhat unusual combination of having high levels of both negative emotionality *and* extraversion/surgency (remember, they usually move in opposite directions) coupled with lower levels of effortful control. This high level of both negative emotionality and extraversion can set up a kind of push–pull phenomenon in which these children are drawn to situations that they can have trouble handling. The lower effortful control also means that these tendencies and emotions are more difficult to control. In many ways, these are the children that Chess and Thomas labeled as "difficult" and others have described as undercontrolled, disengaged, or even "feisty."

4. *Mellow.* The mellow children, like the anxious ones, also tend to be lower in extraversion/surgency but, unlike the anxious children, have lower levels of negative emotionality. They may not rush in to approach a new toy that has lots of bells and whistles but, at the same time, aren't particularly concerned about it either. These children often seem content doing relatively quiet things and sometimes seem to need a little extra help in the motivation category. Many mellow children might have been called "easy" according to the Chess and Thomas framework. From our previous study, they might have been categorized into the "steady" group.

5. *Moderate.* The moderate category is a bit of a catch-all, describing children who don't have extreme levels of any of the major dimensions. This designation in no way implies that these children will be "average" in terms of overall potential or success but simply that the levels of negative emotionality, extraversion, and effortful control are all mid-range in amplitude.

## Your Child's Own Temperament

With those basics in mind, you can now attempt to apply these dimensions and categories to specific people. Figuring out where a child fits along these different dimensions and types is not always easy to do, especially if there aren't a lot of other similarly aged kids running and crawling around to use as a reference. There also may be a tendency to avoid thinking of a particular child as average in any particular trait, à la a Lake Wobegon effect. Then there is the challenge that there are inevitably going to be those kids whose behavior won't fit neatly into any of the designated categories even when rated by experienced child observers. Maybe this child has a unique combination of really low levels of negative emotionality and very average levels of extraversion, for example. Not to worry. The brain, after all, really couldn't care less about the little names that we give things and argue over at scientific conferences. There will always be plenty of folks who defy the tidy boxes that we have so carefully created.

These challenges notwithstanding, this might be a good moment to stop and think about any particular children you might be reading this book for and where that person should be placed along the three main dimensions and five principle types. While there are a number of research-based rating scales that you could complete to do this task officially, a decent estimate can probably be made simply by spending some time considering how your child's behavior compares to similarly aged boys or girls along these core dimensions of temperament. Table 2.1 provides a guide to do this, using the framework proposed by Rothbart.

*Here are the instructions.*   Look at the accompanying table and think about your child's temperament relative to other children of the same gender and age. Use the anchoring statements at either end of the scale to decide upon the best overall number for that child regarding levels of negative emotionality, extraversion, and effortful control. Once you've arrived at a number, categorize it as being low, average, or high according to the following rules. Scores of 1 or 2 are considered low, scores between 3 and 5 are categorized as moderate, and scores of 6 and 7 are recorded as high. Then, based on these categorizations, place the child's temperament into one of the five types as described in Table 2.2.

If there is not an exact match based on the child's individual profile, select the closest one. As you continue reading, keep your child's temperament type in mind as we'll be referring to it in discussions about how the best parental approach might change according to these different types.

If there is another parent, caretaker, or really any other person who knows the child well, it can be an interesting, and sometimes illuminating, exercise to see how much agreement there is with that other person. For a whole host of reasons, we might expect a fair amount of discrepancy between your assessment and that other person's. This doesn't necessarily mean that somebody is wrong

**Table 2.1** A Brief Temperament Rating Scale

| | LOW | | | AVERAGE | | HIGH | | |
|---|---|---|---|---|---|---|---|---|
| | 1 Very low | 2 Low | 3 Slightly low | 4 About average | 5 Slightly high | 6 High | 7 Very high | |
| Low negative emotionality<br>• Rarely angry<br>• Comfortable and adaptable to new situations<br>• Infrequently sad, even-keeled<br>• Takes a lot to make scared or nervous<br>• Rapidly soothed by others | 1 Very low | 2 Low | 3 Slightly low | 4 About average | 5 Slightly high | 6 High | 7 Very high | High negative emotionality<br>• Experiences anger quickly and with high intensity<br>• Quite uncomfortable in many situations<br>• Often sad, upset, and cries easily<br>• Fearful and nervous<br>• Not easily soothed by others |
| Low extraversion<br>• Low energy and less active<br>• Avoids high-stimulation activities<br>• Not impulsive<br>• Often shy around people | 1 Very low | 2 Low | 3 Slightly low | 4 About average | 5 Slightly high | 6 High | 7 Very high | High extraversion<br>• Lots of energy and activity<br>• Seeks out and enjoys high-stimulation activities<br>• Impulsive<br>• Not shy around people |
| Low effortful control<br>• Struggles to focus and concentrate<br>• Unable to delay gratification<br>• Dislikes and avoids quiet activities<br>• Oblivious to changes in environment | 1 Very low | 2 Low | 3 Slightly low | 4 About average | 5 Slightly high | 6 High | 7 Very high | High effortful control<br>• Strong ability to focus and concentrate<br>• Often able to delay gratification<br>• Enjoys and prefers quiet activities<br>• Notices small changes in environment |

Developed by the author based on the model by Rothbart and colleagues.

**Table 2.2** Five Different Temperament Types Based on Levels of the Three Core Dimensions

| Temperament Type | Negative Emotionality | Extraversion | Effortful Control |
|---|---|---|---|
| Moderate | Average | Average | Average |
| Vigorous | Low | High | Average or high |
| Anxious | High | Low | Average or low |
| Agitated | High | High | Low |
| Mellow | Low or average | Low | Average |

or inaccurate, although it might. More often, however, a child's behavior, even those components that we define as core temperament, will actually change in the presence of different contexts or people. This interesting wrinkle in child temperament and a few other important features will be addressed soon.

## Rating Temperament: An Example

If you're struggling a bit to do this exercise, the following example might help.

Three-year-old Lucy lives with her mother and father and recently began attending a local preschool. She is kind and quite obedient, with her teachers saying that she almost always follows the rules. With her parents and when one on one with friends, she is warm and affectionate, but she can struggle when there are bigger groups or new things to try. At birthday parties, she is often quiet and will sometimes claim that she doesn't want to go to the party at all. Her parents also sometimes get frustrated with her reticence to explore or do things on her own without them. At night, Lucy often voices fears about monsters or strange noises, which will frequently cause her to want to sleep in her parents' bed.

With this admittedly limited information, Lucy seems like she might score about a 6 (high) for negative emotionality, given her increased tendency relative to other kids at getting nervous. Her extraversion score might be around 3 based on a lack of interest in high stimulation activities, although not too low as she does enjoy friends and can brighten around her parents. She does seem to show at least average levels of effortful control based on her behavior at school. Putting this profile of high negative emotionality, low extraversion, and average effortful control, Lucy might best be described as being in the anxious group.

## Parent Temperament Matters Too

Like eating certain potato chips, it can be tough when appraising another person's temperament to stop at just one. If, having done the exercise of trying to estimate your child's temperament, you find yourself moving on to your partner, best friend, boss, and of course, yourself, you are not alone. This is a good thing, and I encourage you to repeat the same process for yourself by following the same steps.

Just as certain parenting approaches will be received more or less easily based on the child's temperament, the same is true for parents. In thinking of a more anxious child who could benefit from being supportively "nudged" a bit to confront things that make her a little nervous, for example, that nudging will probably come a lot easier to the parent who isn't highly anxious herself. At the same time, it is also possible that the anxious parent may be more able to empathize with their anxious child about her struggles, while the naturally bold parent might become quickly critical and frustrated.

This is why knowing what you "should" do is often not enough and why an understanding of your own temperament and your own predispositions as a parent can be valuable. In some cases, the science may make a strong case that, in your particular family, a new approach is needed, but that approach runs squarely against the grain of your personality. Maybe, for example, you'll realize after reading the next chapter that your more authoritarian style of parenting doesn't mesh so great with your more agitated-type child, but that style of parenting is what feels most natural to you. In this case, you might need to work on a process I often refer to as parenting "overrides." In so doing, we recognize the fact that changing parental course in a certain way may be important but will certainly not come easily and could likely require additional time or resources. In other instances, of course, parents may find that what is called for fits their natural tendencies just fine or that the level of scientific evidence just isn't compelling enough to warrant a parent trying to swim against the tide of her own personality in the first place. Positive parenting energy, after all, is a finite and precious commodity in the harried world of raising children and needs to be spent wisely.

The pioneering researchers Chess and Thomas not only helped reawaken the concept of temperament but also were responsible for one of the cornerstone theories of child development, namely, the idea of goodness of fit.[13] The main principle here is that temperament traits are not, in and of themselves, positive or negative but instead are more or less adaptable based on how well they *fit* with a particular environment. That environment, in turn, often has a lot to do with the parent's own temperament and personality traits. In thinking of a highly energetic and exuberant child, for example, one could envision that those qualities might work quite well with similarly energetic parents or a teacher who employs a more active style of teaching. The same disposition, however, could cause conflict with parents whose temperament is more in keeping with the mellow type or an "old school" teacher who expects her students to sit quietly during long periods of instruction. In other instances, what may be the most optimal fit is not an environment whose characteristics *match* the child but one that provides a more *complementary* quality. An especially irritable toddler will be a challenge for most households, but when the parents are also prone to have short fuses, the fit could be especially poor, even dangerous.

How do you think your child's temperament fits with your own temperament, or your partner's if you are co-parenting? Are there places where the fit seems especially complimentary or problematic? Often there can be a mix of both, and being aware of these potential trouble spots is a big first step in navigating through these waters. As we begin looking at specific parenting challenges and topics such as screen time and corporal punishment, one important question we'll examine is whether the overall science-based conclusion regarding what is "best" for children might need a little tweaking based on the child or parent's temperament, or other factors. In some cases, we'll find that the general recommendation doesn't deviate much between kids with different temperaments while for other issues it matters a great deal. In still other cases, we'll see that "it depends" factors are important but have little or nothing to do with temperament.

## Fun Facts About Temperament

### Sex and Gender Differences

People love thinking and talking about differences between males and females, but the available science often isn't quite as flashy as the interplanetary differences that some authors espouse.[14] Before getting into all this, it is worth the reminder that the terms *sex* and *gender* denote different things. An individual's sex pertains to one's chromosomes (either XX or XY for the most part) and male–female differences in anatomy, both on the inside and on the outside. *Gender* is a somewhat more difficult term to define but refers more to the thoughts, feelings, and behaviors that have culturally been associated with either sex. It can also relate to a person's inner sense of being male, female, or somewhere in between regardless of genetics or body parts.

Chapter 7 will go into a lot more detail about the process by which young children begin to understand and accept the concept of sex and gender and the degree to which parents can influence that learning. For the sake of this section, however, we will allow for a certain amount of imprecision by having the terms be somewhat synonymous. On most of the temperament questionnaires, after all, parents simply check off a box for male or female with no explanation of what this does and does not mean.

For infants, one area that shows some consistent differences between boys and girls is in activity level, a component of extraversion/surgency. Other than that, however, there isn't much to find.[15] As children get into the preschool years, girls tend to show higher average levels of effortful control with regard to things like maintaining attention and focus a little longer, particularly for lower-stimulation activities. They also tend to be drawn to play activities that involve a little less commotion. These differences likely reflect both genetically influenced predispositions and emerging effects of learning and culture. The magnitudes of these sex differences, however, are not as large as many people expect. If you're at a birthday party with a bunch of 5-year-olds and the crowd suddenly breaks into a full-volume race car, monster truck, demolition derby, chances are that the stars of the show will be a mixed group of boys and girls, as will be the kids watching the performance intently from the sidelines.

When it comes to levels of negative emotionality in younger children, few sex differences tend to be found. This statement may be a surprise to some people because it is fairly well-known that the rates of conditions like anxiety disorders and depression (which have been linked to the trait of negative emotionality) tend to be higher for females compared to males, but these differences are present only from adolescence onward.[16] These observations support the idea that temperament, although important, is not the only cause of these clinical disorders and their increased susceptibilities to girls and women. Life events, hormonal changes, sexism, and many other factors are thought to play key roles in how temperamental traits like negative emotionality lead to clinical disorders like depression in some people but not others.

## Different Kids in Different Situations

As you may have encountered in the previous exercise, summarizing a child's temperament will come easily when thinking about some kids, but for others it will prove more challenging. The latter could happen because the individual possesses one of those more unique profiles that isn't well captured by one of the five categories. It also can occur because it is a little harder to visualize what people look like who possess average levels of traits. Describing someone who is extremely high in extraversion is not that tough, but what does the kid who scores in the 50th percentile of extraversion look like? Making matters even more complicated, there could be two different routes to scoring in the average range on a temperamental trait. First, a child could display very moderate and developmentally expected levels of a trait consistently across time and situations. Alternatively, however, there can also be the child who shows very high levels of a trait in some instances and very low levels in others. A young child might, for example, show marked distress and anxiety in the presence of dogs and thunderstorms but be absolutely fearless when it comes to having new children or teachers at his daycare. In my own practice, I have treated several kids with severe anxiety who had absolutely no problem doing things that would completely terrify most others (including me), like ski jumping. When it comes to scoring these kids on their level of negative emotionality, what is a parent supposed to do with this inconsistency? Simply splitting the difference to settle at some ho-hum average score seems to miss the essence of things here.

Just the idea of a trait being markedly different from moment to moment or from situation to situation seems counterintuitive to the whole idea of what temperament is supposed to be about. By definition, temperament is described as one's *typical* pattern of behavior, but what if a child's normal approach or response to the world is inconsistent and varies a lot based upon the people around her, the time of day, the lunar calendar, or from some unseen factor that nobody has figured out yet?

Lots of moms and dads scratch their heads when, for example, their 2-year-old son throws a fit over being "encouraged" to eat some peas at home but then the next day at grandma's house devours a full meal of foods he has never ever tried in his life. They wonder, "What the heck am I doing (or is grandma doing) differently that is creating this completely different kid?" It could all be a total crapshoot or the random variation of the gods, or there might be something to understand here about parenting style or other factors that cause what are supposed to be fairly fixed patterns of behavior to change dramatically under certain conditions. Science is starting to give this important issue more attention, but much continues to be poorly understood. Ironically, it is possible that temperamental variability may be kind of a trait in and of itself, meaning that some kids have a natural tendency to act pretty much the same wherever they are while others are more reactive to qualities of the environment.

## What Causes Temperament?

There isn't enough room here to launch into a full overview of the many causes of personality and temperament. Nevertheless, some discussion is needed, especially given the relevance of child temperament to parenting. One good place to start might be to explain what temperament is *not*, namely, the pure genetic component of personality. This, unfortunately, is often how temperament gets portrayed, even in some scientific journal articles, but it simply isn't true. Study after study, often using samples of twins, repeatedly shows that genetics and the environment contribute roughly equally to temperament traits, even at very early ages.[17] Infant social smiling is one good example. These wonderful little moments can begin as early as 1 month of age (the grandmother lobby has definitively concluded that any smile before that age is due to gas). Given how young that is, one might logically assume that something like this *has* to be under tight uncontaminated genetic control. However, research has shown strong environmental influences on infant smiling,[18] likely having a lot to do with how much parents and other adults are smiling *at them*. The number of smiles a baby makes seems to be related to the number of smiles a baby takes, in a slight twist from the famous Paul McCartney line.

Genetics is certainly a powerful force when it comes to child temperament, but it gets mixed and even modified through a number of other factors, including the prenatal environment, early experience (good and bad), siblings and peers, levels of stress, and many other factors.[19] Indeed, one of the forces that shape a child's temperament is, actually, parenting. Yes, this is a book that addresses how child temperament may alter the effectiveness and impact of various parenting strategies, but we can't ignore the fact that things can work in the other direction too.[20]

For decades, the old nature–nurture debate trudged on as people argued over the pre-eminence of genetic versus environmental factors as the main driving force behind human behavior. The many previously mentioned twin studies did much to demonstrate that both genetics *and* the environment play strong roles in determining the level of personality and temperament traits.[17,21] After this polite acknowledgment, however, the really interesting research began to emerge showing not only that both genetics and environmental factors were important but that these two conceptually distinct domains were actually interrelated.[22] Genes, it turns out, through a process called gene–environment correlations, seem to have the ability to make certain events more likely to occur by *evoking* particular characteristics of an environment (think how a temperamentally irritable child might pull out more hostile responses from others) or through *actively choosing* one environment over another (think how genetically influenced thrill-seeking behavior might cause a person to hang out with similarly minded friends to form a sky diving club). Another line of research demonstrated that, in many situations, the effect of genes *depends* on the presence of certain environments and the effect of certain environmental factors depends on the presence of certain genes in processes called gene–environment interactions.[23,24] Finally, in an emerging field called epigenetics, it is being increasingly appreciated that while environmental events cannot directly change one's genetic code, they can change the degree to which certain genes are or are not expressed. Through processes such as DNA methylation,[25] in which a carbon atom bonded with three hydrogen atoms attaches itself to a DNA strand and alters a gene's ability to make the encoded protein, genetic expression can be modified, even silenced. In thinking about these fascinating and important mechanisms, the tired nature versus nurture question on many levels ceases even to make sense.

## Implications for Parenting

Before getting too bogged down with the science of child temperament, it might be good at this point to remember why we are bothering to go to the trouble of learning all this stuff about temperament in the first place in this book about parenting. The reason, of course, is the central premise that *the optimal parenting strategy regarding many of the longstanding controversies in parenting is not the same for everyone and may depend on factors like a child's temperament.* In the course of understanding an individual child's temperament more fully and gaining a better appreciation of how temperament or other variables might (or might not) impact key decisions that need to be made, parents can be empowered to make the *best* choices for their *individual* child based on the most *updated evidence-based knowledge.*

My timing in trying to offer evidence for this core hypothesis could not have been luckier. As this chapter was being written, one of the most comprehensive studies on the subject ever done was just published.[26] Combining data across 84 individual research studies, the main finding from this ambitious study was that indeed certain temperamental traits and types do appear to make children more susceptible to parenting behavior "for better or for worse." Specifically, children with more difficult or challenging temperaments, such as those in the agitated category, tend to *benefit the most* from positive parental behavior (things like warmth and providing good limits and monitoring) while at the same time *are most adversely affected* by negative parental behavior (being inconsistent and using harsh discipline). For the mother or father with a temperamentally challenging child, no pressure there! Parenting still mattered for children with less extreme or easier temperaments, just not to the same extent.

At the same time, however, the study also found areas where certain child temperament traits, like extraversion, didn't seem to alter the relation much between positive or negative parenting and later child adjustment. Putting all of this together, we cannot simply assume that child temperament will always throw a huge "it depends" into the best answer to a classic parenting dilemma, but chances are there will be many occasions when it needs to be taken into account.

Keep in mind that this important study looked at parenting and child behavior in very broad strokes by lumping parenting behavior as being overall positive or negative. This book, by contrast, will attempt to drill down to a much more specific level in looking at *particular* parenting controversies and their relations to *specific* temperamental traits and types. Yes, good parenting is good, but that knowledge does not easily translate into the very real 2-AM decision a mother or father needs to make about whether or not to pick up a crying baby for the third time tonight versus giving him 5 minutes on his own to see if he can settle himself down. The following chapters will each endeavor to summarize what science actually knows in general about very specific parenting controversies before picking that answer apart based on who the child is, who the parent is, and other important factors that need to be considered. In some cases, we'll see evidence that certain parenting behavior tends to have similar effects on all types of kids. In other cases, the "correct" science-based answer may depend almost completely on other things. Still, in other cases, the jury with regard to scientific evidence may either still be out or was never summoned in the first place. Sure, it would be wonderful if the answers we sought to parenting's most perennial and vexing controversies could be fully and accurately explained in a 10-second sound bite, but that unfortunately is not the world we live in. We are, after all, talking about the living human brain.

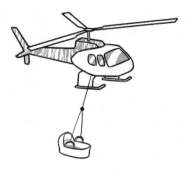

# 3

# Tiger/Attachment/Helicopter Parenting

## Searching for Truth Among the Books and the Blogs

Parents and childcare experts alike often enjoy saying that "there are no manuals for raising children." The truth, however, is that we are bombarded by them. A quick Google search or trip to the bookstore rapidly reveals an overwhelming number of resources that are available to teach you how to raise a happy, confident, empathic, resilient, responsible, (etc.) child. Many guides also exist offering step-by-step instructions for working with more explosive, spirited, strong-willed, or anxious children. Perhaps the most well-known books, however, are those that describe a more all-encompassing approach to parenting, often designed to overcome certain societal trends that are viewed as making the current crop of youth less ideal than previous generations. One justification for there being so many of these books is that they typically don't agree with each other—at all. As Leonard Sax's *Collapse of Parenting*, for example, laments the loss of parental control in today's households,[1] Vicki Hoefle's *Duct Tape Parenting* advocates for 6-year-olds being able to set their own bedtime.[2] Meanwhile, Amy Chua's *Battle Hymn of the Tiger Mother* provides a strong retort to the Western self-esteem movement to nurture and cultivate a child's sense of individuality and specialness.[3]

When immersed in each of these books individually, most all of them seem to make a lot of sense. References to some scientific studies, or at least well-chosen national statistics, are commonly invoked to support the author's central thesis, but contradictory data are generally ignored rather than explained. As for hard evidence that one method is actually superior to others and reliably produces the

Chapter illustrations drawn by Jaq Fagnant

*Parenting Made Complicated.* David C. Rettew, Oxford University Press (2021). © Oxford University Press.
DOI: 10.1093/oso/9780197550977.003.0003

desired final product, this tends to be quite sparse other than some reassurances that the author's own kids turned out okay.

One also gets the feeling while reading popular parenting books that the approaches and strategies that are recommended reflect intellectual justifications of methods that already came naturally to the author, based on his or her own personality. Cognitive psychology research confirms that as much as we'd like to think that our behavior follows from our well-earned beliefs, it often works in the exact reverse. A parent who tends to be more irritable and critical is likely to be drawn to material suggesting that effusive praising of children is overrated, while a parent who tends to be bold and independent is likely to find arguments for free-range parenting to be quite compelling. Such biases don't necessarily negate the points being made in favor of a particular parenting style but should perhaps cause us all to step back and consider which "choir" we belong to and which preacher is going to sound most appealing. The point here is not to psychoanalyze the authors of popular parenting books, but rather for you to be able to take the insights learned in chapter 2 about temperament and apply them toward an honest and objective appraisal of how your own traits are going to affect your behaviors and attitudes on parenting.

## Five Parental Styles

Similar to food diets, it seems like everyone who writes a book or goes on a speaking tour comes up with their own brand and title for their parenting approach. With each one claiming to be new and different, the challenge is in figuring out how the dozens if not hundreds of named parenting styles actually differ from each other. Many share a number of common elements with differences often being more a function of emphasis (or just pure lingo), but at the same time there clearly are many points of divergence where one approach zigs and another zags. With that in mind, the following are five parenting styles that have received a fair amount of attention and media coverage as they compete for the maximum market share of parental energy. Based on well-known books or other colloquial phrases, they will be referred to as (i) intensive (helicopter), (ii) attachment, (iii) old school, (iv) tiger, and (v) free-range.

## Intensive (Helicopter) Parenting

In its more extreme form, intensive parenting (also known as directive or even child-centered parenting) is more commonly known as helicopter or snowplow parenting, although these latter terms are more derogatory and generally used by proponents of *other* approaches. There are few card-carrying mothers and fathers out there who proudly self-identify as helicopter parents. There is also arguably no major figure or book that can be pointed to as the exemplar of the intensive parenting "movement," although a defense by two economists has recently made the scene.[4] Despite the lack of celebrity endorsements, however, it is probably fair to say that intensive parenting is the signature approach of our times and the default parenting framework especially for progressively minded white middle- and upper-class families in the United States.[5] These characteristics also make it the punching bag for advocates of other types of parenting styles.

While there is no standard definition of intensive parenting, it generally describes a style in which parents are quite actively involved in the parenting process as they try to cultivate a child-rearing environment that is positive, successful, fun, growth-promoting, and not overly stressful. Intensive parents *get involved* in their child's life: they get themselves down on the floor and are willing to play Candyland seven times in a row if requested. And when their kids are being cared for by others, intensive parents are not afraid to engage neighbors, teachers, coaches, and other adults to ensure that their child experiences a similar environment in other settings. Intensive parents tend to be generous with their praise in an effort to build self-esteem and try to avoid overly harsh and critical language. They also often subscribe to the idea that "kids should be kids," which means providing a fair amount of protection from potential threats, lots of structured activity options, and a lot of direct assistance to children when needed. In contrast to some of the other approaches, intensive parents are more willing to jump in and rescue children when they are struggling or even likely to struggle.

One day many years ago, I was fortunate to have two psychiatrists from Bali join me as I saw patients in my clinic. With a family's permission we would see patients and parents together, and between appointments we would comment on our observations. After seeing a child who had been diagnosed with attention-deficit/hyperactivity disorder and who couldn't stay still for more than 10 seconds, I asked the young doctors if that was behavior they saw in Bali. Oh, yes, they replied. We then saw another family who left the appointment in a bit of a hurry after the parents helped the child open my large and somewhat tricky door to get out. One of the doctors then made a comment that showed that he was noticing things I had missed by pointing out that in Bali, the parents would have patiently waited several minutes for the child to open the door herself. This was a subtle but very illustrative example of intensive parenting.

The principles of intensive parenting often seems to be reinforced by schools, popular media, and much of the conventional wisdom from child development experts. At the same time, however, intensive parenting is frequently ridiculed (hence the helicopter and snowplow terms) as being too willing to do things that children should be expected to do themselves and too shielding of anything in the big bad world that might cause a young child fear or distress. Thus, a major criticism of the intensive or helicopter parenting style is that it fails to promote the grit, perseverance, and toughness required to succeed as an independent adult and instead produces more emotionally fragile individuals who lack many basic skills of daily living.

## Attachment Parenting

The attachment parenting approach focuses on methods, particularly when children are very young, that are designed to cultivate a child's inner sense of security and connectedness. This parenting style emphasizes warmth and attunement while actively avoiding methods seen as harsh or insensitive, such as corporal punishment.

One aspect of attachment parenting that can be confusing is the difference between it and the overall concept of attachment. Beginning with notable figures such as British psychiatrist John Bowlby in the 1950s and 1960s, who worked with children in England during the turmoil of World War II, there has been an increasing appreciation of the impact of early stress and parental separation on child development. While this may seem pretty obvious now, psychiatrists up until then often focused more on a young child's *fantasy* environment than his or her *actual* environment. In 1965, a student of Bowlby, Mary Ainsworth, developed a laboratory protocol called the Strange Situation to measure the strength of the bond between an infant (usually at around 15 months of age) and a parent. This procedure, still used today, involves a series of maneuvers in which a parent is in the room with their child when a friendly stranger joins the mix.[6] The mother then leaves the room briefly and then returns. All the while, observers code how the child reacts to the stranger, the separation, and, most important, what happens when the parent reunites with the infant. "Securely" attached infants definitely tend to notice that the mother has left the room and express their unhappiness about it, but when the mother returns they soothe quickly and return to their baseline. Insecurely attached infants can show different patterns such as remaining very angry and upset after reunification, to looking like they couldn't care less that the mother is gone, to disorganized and chaotic behavior that doesn't fit any pattern at all. These different styles of attachment behavior have been theorized to be the result of how well a parent has done in terms of responding consistently and sensitively to the needs of the baby.

From this fairly humble procedure, there has been a mountain of research basically demonstrating that infants who show secure attachment patterns do better in life than insecurely attached infants on a whole host of outcomes including future mental health, academic achievement, and overall functioning.[7,8] While there has certainly been some evidence that attachment status is more of a two-way street than originally conceptualized, with a child's temperament and genetics playing a role,[9] the scientific literature on attachment status overall is well respected and continues to be very influential.

Attachment parenting arose from these principles and research findings as a strategy parents could take to promote this strong bond that appears so important for future well-being. The actual term was coined by husband-and-wife, pediatrician-and-nurse team William and Martha Sears in 2001 with their book, *The Attachment Parenting Book*.[10] From these ideas and publications, attachment parenting has developed into the enterprise that it is today. Indeed, it is probably fair to say that compared to the other global parenting styles, the attachment parenting approach is the most organized and visible—complete with official organizations such as Attachment Parenting International, conferences that people can attend, and even their own academic journal.

One of the core ideas is that a strong initial attachment bond helps create a "secure base," which gets internalized by the child and thus actually promotes *more* independence and exploration later in life. Establishing this strong connection is accomplished by paying attention to the four Bs, namely bonding, babywearing, breastfeeding, and boundary building.[11] A more recent book called *Attached to the Heart* outlines eight core principles of attachment parenting, which also include things such as providing consistent and loving care and balancing personal and family life.[12]

Advocates of attachment parenting have often been vocal in their opposition to many common parenting practices such as having infants sleep on their own as well as disciplinary methods such as spanking and even time-outs. In their defense, attachment parenting promoters often point to the vast amount of data that exist for humans and animals alike demonstrating how important a strong attachment bond is for future health and the negative effects that can occur when early relationships are disrupted or abusive.

The critics of attachment parenting, and there are many, cite a number of frustrations and concerns. These include the promotion of co-sleeping with infants, despite evidence that doing so may increase the risk of suffocation, and what many consider to be their overzealous and scientifically unsupported attacks on parenting techniques such as ignoring and time-outs. The science behind both sleep training methods and disciplinary methods are given their own chapter later in this book. Another major critique of attachment parenting, especially from those supportive of the old school approach described next, is that it is overly indulgent and may lead to helicopter parenting and a general spoiling of a child, a charge that makes most attachment parenting advocates bristle. Opponents of attachment parenting further maintain that the scientific evidence for attachment per se should not be usurped and extrapolated as endorsements for attachment parenting, which has not been directly studied to anywhere near the same level. Relatedly, critics also point out that some of the core principles of attachment parenting, such as being loving and consistent, are really pretty universal values that have more to do with common sense than any particular parenting modality.

## Old School Parenting

The old school parent often yearns for the good old days of yesteryear, when children weren't "coddled" and a smart mouth was dealt with by a swift smack on the behind. This parenting style is not a democracy. The parents are the bosses, and their rule is not to be questioned or challenged. Values that are important to the old school parent include respect for authority (especially the parents themselves), hard work, and emotional toughness. Rather than children being encouraged to discuss more vulnerable feelings, these kids may get told, "Don't cry or I'll give you something to cry about." Ideally, however, these children also understand that this tougher approach is being done for their own good and feel secure in knowing that there are responsible adults imposing reasonable limits on their behavior. As such, these children are able to develop close family bonds with both parents and siblings. In the practice of parents not always putting the needs of the child above everything else, a child is also thought to learn essential lessons in humility, sacrifice, and collaboration within groups.

While the parenting style for old school parents would often be labeled as "strict," there often are many opportunities for independence. Old school parents don't hover and thus allow children to explore the world on their own and be exposed to "adult" things earlier in life. While an intensive parent and an old school parent might each take a young child fishing, the intensive parent throws the fish back while the child of the old school parents is pushed to scale, clean, and eat the fish for dinner.

A recent homage to old school parenting was written by family physician and psychologist Leonard Sax in his book *The Collapse of Parenting*. In this work, he laments the world of intensive parenting where mothers and fathers are reduced to negotiators and cajolers, trying to get their children just to swallow three bites of peas for dinner. He traces recent trends in psychiatric medication usage and obesity in children to the destruction of a more hierarchically oriented family structure in which children did what they were told to do without parents needing to provide a dissertation as to the reasons.

It is easy for many adults to feel a little nostalgic for old school parenting. However, critics readily point to the slippery slope that can exist between being tough and being abusive and the volumes of data that exist on the negative effects of childhood trauma. Advocates of more intensive parenting tend to roll their eyes when they hear adult children talking about their stereotypical old school fathers who loved them even though they never showed it.

## Tiger Parenting

The term *tiger parenting* comes directly from the bestselling book by attorney Amy Chua called *Battle Hymn of the Tiger Mother*, which was published in 2011 and described her own parenting model based on what she experienced as a child. It describes an approach in which parents actively push their children to work hard and be successful. Parents can be strict and, at times, critical but are also extremely supportive and involved with their children. Rules and prohibitions are many, and family life is highly valued.

While the book references the popularity of the approach among families from countries such as China, Japan, and India, it is certainly present in families across cultures, and is not as ubiquitous among Asian American families as is often believed.[13] Indeed, lest we fall into overly stereotypical beliefs about parenting style and cultural background, a direct challenge to tiger parenting was described in the book *Dolphin Parenting, A Parent's Guide to Raising Happy, Healthy, and Motivated Children Without Turning Into a Tiger*, written by child psychiatrist Shimi Kang, who advocates for a less pressured and more playful approach that she experienced from her own India-born parents.[14]

To be fair, *Tiger Mother* is actually not an unequivocal endorsement of this particular approach but rather a memoir that shows quite a bit of self-introspection, nondogmatic thinking, and, actually, humor. Nevertheless, the book became a kind of cultural icon, drawing both fans and critics, the latter of which often voiced concern that tiger parenting could lead to outwardly successful individuals who were anxious and never satisfied that their considerable accomplishments were good enough.

The tiger parent approach has some similarities with the old school style. Both styles demand respect from children and discourage large amounts of "down time" for kids to do with as they please. With tiger parenting, however, a greater emphasis is placed on setting high expectations in areas such as academic achievement, sports accomplishments, and musical proficiency and then enforcing arduous homework and practice schedules to ensure that these expectations are met. By contrast, old school parents may be a little more likely to push kids to do more mundane chores at home even if that might cut into time otherwise spent engaging in loftier pursuits. The degree of prohibition against things like playdates, sleepovers, or watching television is also often at a level that might exceed what would be encountered with an old school parent (although nobody is really keeping track of these rules).

Some similarities further exist between tiger and intensive parents. Both tiger and intensive parents might well be expected to put the kibosh on, for example, a 5-year-old child who wants to spend a few hours in the woods to build a fort out of sticks, but the intensive (aka helicopter) parent would do so out of safety concerns whereas the tiger parent might consider it a waste of time. Tiger parenting in younger children would include more of things like starting music lessons and beginning basic arithmetic drills at an early age and less of things like having a parent sit down on the floor for a child-led play session. Praise and compliments among tiger parents would also be less abundant under the idea that a child's self-esteem is not something that can be given by someone else but rather needs to be earned through genuine success and hard work.

## Free-Range Parenting

In many ways, the free-range parenting approach stands apart from the others in its strong recommendation for parents to basically back off. When many parents think back to their own childhood, what often comes to mind is being given a fair amount of space in which to ramble and explore on their own. Growing up in a relatively safe southern New Jersey suburb, I spent much of my considerable unscheduled time during my elementary school years largely free to roam about a square mile of neighborhood that included several friend's houses, a stream, a lake, and a number of busy roads, without the need to inform my parents about where exactly I was (provided I got home for dinner by 6 PM). This arrangement led to more than few instances of bullying and being the target of diabolical plots from the older crowd with which I tended to associate, but for the most part I thrived and greatly benefited from the confidence that such an arrangement provided me.

Compare that now with the much more controlled and supervised system of today, in which many parents expect and demand to know where their kids are at all times (if not being able to just look on their smartphone) and in which playdates are arranged and usually prepared for well in advance. To some, this shift toward intensive or helicopter parenting comes at a big price with kids becoming more and more anxious and ill-prepared for a world that they now experience (at least first-hand) less and less. What's more, the spoon-feeding that intensive parents are providing deprives children of important opportunities to learn self-reliance and gain confidence in their ability to follow their passion and overcome obstacles with perseverance and hard work, a critical skill that psychologist Angela Duckworth has called "grit."[15]

Thus, the momentum for free-range parenting comes in direct response to the intensive or helicopter style. It emphasizes some aspects of old school parenting while being less concerned with kids needing to learn their place as subordinates who must be taught to respect authority. Advocates of free-range parenting relish pointing out and make fun of news stories that depict, for example, overly neurotic parents afraid to let their children eat Halloween candy from anyone they don't know, or who call the police after they witness a kindly 80-year-old man talk to their son and pat him on the head at a supermarket, or who wire their healthy infant's room with cameras and sensors able to monitor their baby's every move and vital signs. Advocates also fight back against instances in which the police or child welfare agency intervene with young children whose parents permit them to explore their near surroundings without a chaperone.

The book that coined and really energized this parenting style was called *Free-Range Kids*, written in 2009 by writer and columnist Lenore Skenazy after she received intensely negative media attention for letting her 9-year-old son ride the New York subway on his own.[16] In the book she points out that across many parts of the world the actual instance of many bad things happening to kids has been dropping almost as fast as the parental worry surrounding these bad things has been rising.

The free-range parenting approach is gaining in popularity. In addition to Skenazy's book, there have been many others pushing that parents pull back from overprotecting their children and shielding them from every negative element of society. Recently in 2018, the Utah state legislature actually unanimously passed a law that was known in the media as the "free range parenting bill."[17] It attempted to offer a more restrictive definition of child neglect that purposely excluded things like children of "sufficient age" to do things like walk to school on their own, play outside without direct adult supervision, or go to a store. The new law was purposely vague about what "sufficient age" actually meant. In deliberations over the bill, interestingly, it turned out that the state's child protective services had never actually pressed neglect charges against a parent for something like an unsupervised playground visit, but the legislature was apparently looking to take pre-emptive action.

Critics of free-range parenting, meanwhile, remind parents of the unfortunate and sometimes deadly consequences that can result when children are left to their own devices. Children's brains process risk differently than adults and can underestimate dangers that any quick check of the day's headlines will show are still present. There is also the concern that, for some people, the free-range approach provides some intellectual cover for parents who basically would just rather not be parents at all.

Beyond these five styles, of course, there are many others that often come with their own book and mascot. A quick search online and one can easily learn about elephant, jellyfish, and the previously mentioned dolphin parenting style in addition to lighthouse, holistic, slow, and unconditional approaches. Like the dozens of cereal choices at the grocery store, these models often reflect a different emphasis on a small number of core ingredients. That said, following one approach over another will frequently result in a real and practical difference to the way a parent responds to a common challenging situation, as the next section will demonstrate.

## Parenting Style Differences in Action

To illustrate how these different styles might lead to differences in specific parenting behaviors, consider the following vignette, likely not that uncommon if you have young children.

Jamie is a 5-year-old boy who is watching a video on an iPad. In walks his 3-year-old sister who makes a beeline to a tower that the little boy has recently made with some blocks. She starts pulling on some blocks and the tower partially crumbles. The boy yells at his sister, runs over to her, and yanks a block out of his sister's hand. When she tries to grab it back, he hits her, knocking her to the ground. The mother, who had been preparing a snack for the kids in the kitchen, now comes into the room to find her daughter sitting on the floor crying and her son in full meltdown mode over the fact that his building has been "ruined."

How might the mother respond in this situation according to the principles of these major parenting styles? A mom operating from an intensive or helicopter parenting perspective might try to use one of the techniques she read about online about "giving the toy a time-out" or try to shower concern on the *daughter* so her son realizes that hitting does not gain him additional attention. Most important, though, she is likely to stay in the room and may even act as a physical barrier to prevent the two siblings from interacting for a while. An old school or tiger mother, meanwhile, would be having none of this squabble, and might quickly raise her voice at the son. A spanking here could also be a real possibility for the boy, who is also likely to be told to stop crying over something so small as a few blocks falling on the ground. The free-range mother, by contrast, would be much less likely to get directly involved either as a safety barrier or to dish out a specific punishment, preferring instead to tell them that the blocks belong to both of them and they need to work out how to share them without violence. Finally, the attachment parenting mother might check to make sure the daughter isn't hurt and then crouch down to the level of her son. After assisting him in calming down with some deep breathing, she might tell her son that she understands why he got upset with his tower being demolished but needs to learn how to "use his words" when he gets angry. She might try to facilitate some sort of reconciliation between the siblings, but a specific punishment like a time-out would generally not be given.

In hearing these different responses, you may recognize your own typical reaction to a scenario like this. Or you may recall having mixed and matched many or all of these different methods at various times based on a deliberate choice you made or just your prevailing mood that minute. Or you might be thinking that there isn't enough information in this little vignette to make a good choice (if so, then you are thinking like many scientists). You also might be a little surprised that there are so many potential options out there, many or all of which seem to make at least some sense. As mentioned previously, just the process of moving from parenting reactively to a position of stopping for a second and considering the different options you actually have in the moment can be an extremely large and beneficial step. That said, it would be good to know which approach, if any, is most well supported by the scientific evidence. This is where we head next.

## How the Academics Talk About Parenting

In hearing these descriptions, it can be tempting to reduce each parenting style to a negative caricature of itself—intensive parenting as overprotective, attachment as indulgent, tiger and old school as harsh and insensitive, and free-range as negligent. We see this commonly when advocates of one style quickly try to brush over in blogs or articles the attributes of rival approaches. Yet we also know that there is a lot of subjectivity to words like *strict* or *independent*. Two parents who both see themselves as free-range, for example, may have quite different ideas about what constitutes an acceptable amount of supervision for a 4-year-old. To capture these quantitative differences and to provide some solid evidence to back up the many claims made about the different parenting approaches, it's time to head back into the world of behavioral research.

When we do, we run into a lot of data. However, much of that is targeted not at the more global level of overall parenting style but at particular parenting behaviors that are typically associated with one approach more than others. These might include things like using or not using sleep training methods, corporal punishment, and praise, and each of these topics is covered in detail in upcoming chapters. When it comes to research on the whole enchilada parenting style, we discover that the researchers seem not to have read popular books like *Tiger Mother* or *Free-Range Kids*. Instead, the academic types tend to use a whole different framework to describe the major categories of parenting style.

## Authoritative, Authoritarian, and Permissive Parenting

In the 1970s, psychologist Diana Baumrind proposed a model of understanding parenting styles that was later enhanced by Maccoby and Martin.[18,19] It centered around two critical dimensions of parenting that were initially described as responsiveness and demandingness but are now often referred to as warmth and control. The dimension of warmth relates to how much affection, support, and positivity parents provide to their children while the control dimension pertains to the number of limits and boundaries that are placed on a child and the vigor with which they are monitored and enforced. Both of these domains are very much dimensions, with parents able to be anywhere along the spectrum, but for simplicity sake it is also possible to divide parents as possessing either low or high levels of each of these two dimensions. Putting that in a $2 \times 2$ table then (somewhat artificially) creates four categories of parenting style.

### Authoritative (High Control, High Warmth)
This style of parenting is characterized by parents who both impose reasonable limits and rules for their children but who also are loving and supportive. While these parents often set clear expectations to their children, they are willing to discuss and, at times, modify them. These parents also tend to be quite involved in the task of parenting, which includes proactively supporting their child's reasonable desires for independence.

### Authoritarian (High Control, Low Warmth)
Authoritarian parents also are likely to have a lot of rules and expectations but enforce them somewhat more rigidly. Obedience is expected and demanded without a lot of explanations or, especially, negotiations. The structure of these families tends to be more of dictatorship than a democracy, with the parents knowing what is best and the children expected to fall in line. If they don't, authoritarian parents are likely to dole out stern words and punishments. This is not the style of parenting in which mothers and fathers get accused of acting more like friends to their children then parents. There certainly can be a lot of love in these families, but it often lacks that warm fuzzy quality that might be more evident in authoritative households. Of note, if you are struggling now with the similarity between the words *authoritative* and *authoritarian*, join the club.

### Permissive (Low Control, High Warmth)

Children with permissive parents "enjoy" fewer rules and are less likely to be subjected to punishment when they misbehave. Whether through a deliberate choice or because of the parents' own personalities, conflicts are generally avoided, and these children often have high levels of autonomy. The level of closeness and warmth is high, and there can be a lot of positive interactions between children and parents, but there is much more of a feeling of parents being buddies to their children than authority figures. Children can learn from some of the less optimal choices they make, but it is more likely to come from the natural consequences that ensue more than from any penalties invoked by the parents themselves.

### Uninvolved (Low Control, Low Warmth)

Finally, there is also a fourth group of uninvolved or neglectful parents reflective of both low control and low warmth. As might be expected, however, there aren't too many folks out there championing this particular approach, and at more extreme levels this "style" can drift toward being outright neglectful. Many of these parents are struggling to manage their own hardships and emotional-behavioral challenges. While this group is often associated with families from low socioeconomic backgrounds, it can also arise in wealthy families where parents are more involved in their own pursuits and less interested in the task of raising children.

## Reconciling the Two Frameworks

The disconnect between the academic world's focus on defining parenting style along the authoritative/authoritarian/permissive categories and the intensive/attachment/old school/tiger/free-range (and many other) designations used more commonly in public discourse creates some translation problems. As mentioned, the challenge is not only due to the different terminology but also in the interpretation of what parents are doing. In *Collapse of Parenting*, for example, Sax considers the parenting style he advocates for to be very much an authoritative stance, although others who have reviewed the book put it squarely in the authoritarian camp.[20,21] Similarly, many free-range parents advocates similarly argue that they, of course, believe in reasonable rules and limits but simply define "reasonable" differently than, say, a helicopter parent.[22]

In full realization, then, that we are venturing into some cloudy waters, Figure 3.1 attempts to provide a way to superimpose some of the popular parenting terms onto the scheme used much more commonly in research studies.

When in doubt, I placed each circle closer to how advocates of a particular style would define *itself* rather than how critics of the approach would judge it. In so doing, one thing that becomes immediately evident is that, with the possible

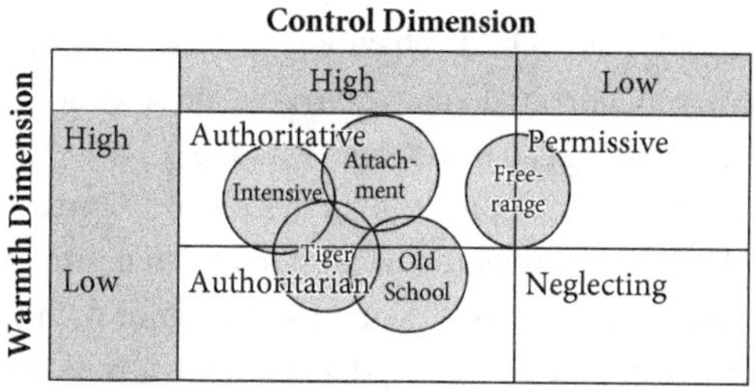

**Figure 3.1** Mapping Popular with Academic Parenting Styles

exception of free-range parenting, all of the major styles cluster in or at least near the high warmth, high control authoritative style. Both intensive and attachment parenting occupy the space most aligned in the authoritarian quadrant with tiger and old school falling lower on the warmth dimension. The size of the individual circles also is a reminder that there can be some variability within each style, just as two people who both call themselves, say, a Republican might have different views on some specific issues.

## Research on Parenting Style

With all of these terms and disclaimers behind us, we can finally look at what science actually knows with regard to which parenting style is best, keeping in mind that what "best" means could mean different things to different people. For some parents, the ultimate goal for their children might be for them to be happy; for others, it is more apt to be defined by achievement and success, and for others still it could be a hope for self-actualization—a child simply being able to live the kind of life that he wants to lead. All of these different outcomes and more have been the target of research studies, and somewhat remarkably, they often converge with regard to their association with parenting style. To cut to the chase, *the research points fairly overwhelmingly toward the conclusion that the authoritative parenting style is related to the most positive outcomes for the greatest number of children.*[23] In many research studies, warmth, positive control, and their combination have been shown to be associated with a large number of generally preferred outcomes such as lower levels of child emotional-behavioral problems, less adolescent substance use, improved academic performance, higher self-esteem, and improved parent–child relationship.[24-27]

An example of the many studies out there is one that looked at a group of 108 African American preschool children and their mothers, about half of whom were parenting on their own.[28] Authoritative parenting was correlated with lower levels of child behavior problems while the authoritarian and permissive styles were correlated with higher levels of child behavioral problems, even after controlling for factors such as family income and education. Another recent study demonstrated just how important parenting can be not only with regard to behavioral outcomes in children but also for brain development. In a sample of 177 Australian adolescents, researchers were able to document the negative effect that growing up from disadvantaged backgrounds can have on the developing brain, such as increased thickness over time of a region called the amygdala that is involved, among other things, in our fear response. Among disadvantaged youth who had experienced more positive (authoritative) parenting, however, the growth of the amygdala over time was attenuated, suggesting that parental warmth and support can partially protect the brain against some of the negative effects of socioeconomic stress.[29]

The skeptics among you might be wondering at this point about how exactly this "just right" goldilocks style of authoritative parenting gets measured by researchers. Most commonly, they just ask, and in doing so often ask only *one* parent about the approach that they presumably apply to *all* of the family's other children. Obviously, this methodology can be problematic as it can potentially lead not only to parents overreporting how awesome they are but also to wide interpretations over what various terms mean. For example, an item from the Parental Authority Questionnaire asks adults to recall the degree to which their parents allowed them to be "free to make up their own minds."[30] To some, such a statement might apply to political beliefs and to others, bedtime. Some research studies also will record a child and parent playing together or working on a particular task and then try to code this interaction along the various parenting dimensions. This method certainly is more objective but suffers both from parents often being on their best behavior and a setting, often in the researcher's lab, that is unnatural for both child and parent.

Further, some research that doesn't assume that parents use the same style for everyone (which is what kids have been protesting for decades) has indeed found that parenting practices can be different between siblings. From our own data, we found that parents report more inconsistent parenting among siblings who meet criteria with attention-deficit/hyperactivity disorder compared to the sibling who does not have that diagnosis, with the hypothesis being that some of these differences are being evoked from the child's behavior.[31] These reasons and others call attention to the need to dig a little deeper before concluding that authoritative parenting is universally the best way to go for everyone.

## It Depends

Parents willing to go beyond soundbites and blog posts on parenting style will quickly find that the actual research literature is full of little holes and inconsistencies that often get glossed over in an effort to arrive at a more global recommendation. Many studies find that the authoritative style seems to work best, but some don't, while others find that it holds only for girls or boys, older kids or younger kids, or for some cultural groups but not others. While often overlooked, it's also common for some of the most notable figures associated with a particular parenting style to have a more nuanced view of their approach than they typically are given credit for by the public. Original tiger mother Amy Chua, for example, is pretty clear in her book that her approach requires some adjustments for particular types of kids, based on her own experience as a mother. Thus, it makes sense to turn to two of the most widely studied "it depends" factors that might indicate the need for some adjustment to the overall recommendation for an authoritative approach to raising children.

## Culture

An important "it depends" factor that is increasingly being recognized is cultural background.[32,33] A recent review of many studies that looked at how the association between parenting style and child success (as measured by academic achievement and level of behavioral problems) found evidence that the superiority of the authoritative style in Western countries was stronger for non-Hispanic white families than in Asian families. While they did not find evidence for one of the other different parenting styles clearly rising to the top for families of non-European decent, the bottom line was that the links between authoritative parenting and good outcomes, as well as more authoritarian and permissive parenting and bad outcomes, were much less clear in these groups.[33]

Studies from families living in other countries also can show more of a mixed bag when it comes to parenting style. In one study from Spain, adolescents assessed across many different domains (self-esteem, behavioral problems, grades, physical health) found associations between better outcomes and both the authoritative and permissive style relative to the authoritarian and, not surprisingly, neglectful approach.[34] From these studies, it appears that it may be necessary to drill down even deeper to the level of the individual child.

## Child Temperament

All this brings us to the radical notion that the optimal parenting style for one child might be at least slightly different from another. While this will certainly strike many parents as something that is inherently obvious, the question is whether or not there is actual scientific evidence to back up this claim. The answer is there is plenty.

Recall from chapter 2 the article that examined 84 individual research studies to see if the association between parenting style and child behavior, cognition, and social ability changed based upon the temperament of the child.[35] Overall, the answer was yes, in that children who were rated as more temperamentally difficult (meaning kids that would likely fall in the agitated or anxious group as described in the chapter) reaped more benefit from positive parenting and suffered more in response to negative parenting relative to temperamentally "easy" children. In doing their analyses, the authors were stuck using the various parenting style definitions of the original studies but noted that in general what they called positive parenting lined up pretty well with the authoritative approach.

As an example, one of the studies in this meta-analysis involving younger children came from the National Institute of Child Health and Human Development Study of Early Child Care and Youth Development, an important project that will be covered in more detail in the daycare versus homecare chapter.[36] Across 10 different locations, over 1000 children and their families were studied from infancy to age 11. Parenting was assessed through observation at home visits, and children were measured across a broad range of domains including academic testing, behavioral problems, and social behavior. The researchers found that more involved, supportive, and responsive parenting predicted better child functioning in all areas, but particularly for the kids who temperamentally were more anxious, more intense, and less inherently adaptable to new places and people. Another study found that among more temperamentally inhibited toddlers, mood and anxiety problems were particularly problematic among children who parents used a more permissive style.[37]

Indeed, there is reason to expect that components of all the major parenting styles, especially in extreme form, can pose some developmental hazards for children who display strong temperament traits. A summary of such hypotheses, many of which unfortunately are still in need of more actual research evidence to confirm these predictions, is found at the end of the chapter. Toddlers and preschoolers who are more anxious, for example, may evoke more overprotective responses in helicopter-style parents which, in turn, can limit a child's opportunities to overcome their fears.[38] At the same time, a more permissive style has also been shown to be associated with increased levels of future anxiety,[37] possibly through parents not engaging in that important nudging that some anxious kids need to get them to take steps they might otherwise not do on their own. Authoritarian or more old school/tiger approaches don't fare any better with anxious kids who often can become even more intimidated and anxious by these domineering parents, but this style could be much less of a problem for kids who temperamentally are more fearless and disinhibited and require a louder "signal" from parents to change their behavior.[39-41]

Similarly, one might also speculate that moving toward more of a free-range approach might benefit kids in the vigorous temperament group who show enough extraversion and surgency to want to explore the world on their own but also sufficient inner caution and self-regulation skills not to take foolish and unnecessary risks. Children in the mellow category, by contrast, may need some of the additional external motivation that is commonly present in more old school- or tiger-leaning parents to propel them to achieve at their maximum potential. These children also tend to be quite happy to sit back and let parents do things *for* them, which can present some challenges for intensive parents with more helicopter tendencies.

## Some Final Strange Sounding Advice

In the end, parents might gain from the recognition that each of the major parenting styles emphasizes something important for child development. The intensive parenting style highlights the fact that raising children requires a real investment in one's time and energy, while attachment parenting helps us remember how beneficial it is to kids when they experience close emotional and physical bonds with trusting adults. Old school parenting, meanwhile, reminds us that our job as parents is not to be our child's best buddy and that sometimes kids need a tougher approach to get on track. Some of these themes are underscored in the tiger parenting style, which also stresses the principle that when you believe your children can succeed then you are more likely to see them rise to their full potential. Finally, free-range parents teach us that, as hard as it may be for parents, children's growth requires them to do things for themselves, on their own—even if it means failing and making bad choices from time to time.

With all this in mind, let me try to offer a simple but perhaps odd sounding piece of advice that pulls all of this science on parenting styles and temperament together: *think about the way that you parent most naturally and then consider taking a deliberate step or two in the* opposite *direction.* I know, I know—this sounds almost diametrically opposite to what legendary parenting experts such as Dr. Spock and others have said about parenting instinctually. And, indeed, that guidance isn't necessarily in conflict with my strange sounding suggestion. Rather, the point here is to be able to recognize that most of us parent in a way that comes most easily to us and, maybe at times, too easily. Very often this can work just fine, but there may be instances when our default mode is a little out of balance. Parents who struggle showing warmth and affection, for example, might do well to make a purposeful effort to be a little more nurturing, while those who naturally feel extremely protective for their kids may need to work on backing off a bit. For most parents, this is not about making a total transformation but rather tweaks that require some conscious effort in order to overcome the momentum of our own temperamental tide.

I actually have tried this myself and found this exercise to be very useful (and hard). Based on my own personality and lifestyle, I've been able to identify, with the help of my wife, that my own natural tendencies can push me to move a little too far into the helicopter arena. Being so busy, it is often much more efficient for me to just take care of things myself rather than letting my kids muddle through various tasks and responsibilities. But this approach robs my kids of the opportunity to learn skills and responsibilities that they will need growing up. I also have recognized that while I tend to admire parents who can show some "tough love" when the situation calls for it, I'm not very good at it, preferring instead to avoid conflict and confrontation. While this quality has provided a large number of very positive interactions with my kids that I truly believe has benefited them (none of them are particularly oppositional or defiant so far, knock on wood), there probably have been a few missed opportunities along the way to help them learn valuable lessons more clearly. Furthermore, my approach may have had more negative consequences if my kids had been more inclined to be more rebellious and less responsible than they are.

These observations bring us back to the very opening sentences of this book. All kids need love. All kids need limits. After that, things can get complicated. This chapter has shown that there is actually quite a bit of science to support that idea that children overall respond best to a parenting style that mixes warmth and support with a level of limits and monitoring that is organizing but not suffocating. The best exact mix of these ingredients is not the same for every child and depends on a number of factors such as the cultural background of the family and the specific temperamental traits of both individual children and parents. Finding that precise sweet spot for your unique family may require thinking beyond the easy but overly prescriptive parenting labels of popular books and blogs. It likely also involves being able to move off of our parental comfort zone as dictated by our own temperament and personal history. Being able to pull these things off is a tall order. Fortunately for us and for our kids, however, perfection here isn't required. And as we now turn to more specific parenting dilemmas and debates that are frequently encountered in the course of a child's early development, we'll do well to keep in mind the value of parenting deliberately, rationally, and flexibly with each new curveball our lives and our children throw at us.

## It Depends—General Parenting Styles

### General Summary

An authoritative parenting style, characterized by firm limits and clear expectations in combination with warmth and support, has been shown to be associated most positively with child development compared to more authoritarian or permissive approaches. In more extreme forms, intensive, attachment, old school, tiger, and free-range parenting styles can be suboptimal for a child's growth, particularly among children with certain temperamental profiles.

| "It Depends" Factor | Adjustment |
| --- | --- |
| Anxious and agitated temperament type | These groups may respond most favorably to an authoritative style that includes warmth and support but also reasonable limits and control while being most susceptible to overly harsh or permissive approaches present in old school or free-range styles. |
| Vigorous type | Often can benefit from being given additional independence (free-range) and responsibility (tiger) if child shows good self-regulation skills |
| Moderate type | Overall somewhat less responsive to parenting style although general principles previously mentioned apply |
| Mellow type | May require additional expectations and motivations (tiger/old school) to achieve at maximum potential |

# PART 2
# INFANCY

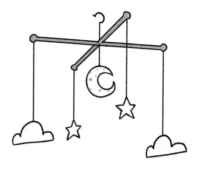

# 4

# Pick Them Up or Let Them Cry (for a While)?

## The Passionate Debate Over Sleep Training

What to do when an infant or toddler repeatedly wakes up crying in the middle of the night is one of the eternal and most passionate debates in parenting. The question is steeped in history, morality, culture, and, sadly, a lot less science than most people expect. Making matters feel even more substantive, this decision about immediately comforting and soothing young children versus employing techniques designed to help them go back to sleep on their own is in many ways the first real intervention designed to *change behavior* that many new moms and dads must choose to undertake . . . or not.

It usually starts innocently enough. Newborns need to eat frequently, and when they are hungry, they really couldn't care less whether you as the parent are twiddling your thumbs with nothing to do, trying to sleep, or watching the start of your favorite show. Parents, usually mothers, then find themselves up every 2 to 4 hours during the newborn period and often for several months after that. When new parents first come up for air and begin to make appearances to the outside world, one of the first questions they usually encounter from sympathetic friends and families is, "How are you sleeping?" The bleary-eyed parents often try to shrug off their fatigue as a rite of passage, even a badge of honor, but research shows that sleep deprivation is no joke for either the parent or the child

Chapter illustrations drawn by Jaq Fagnant

*Parenting Made Complicated.* David C. Rettew, Oxford University Press (2021). © Oxford University Press.
DOI: 10.1093/oso/9780197550977.003.0004

and can lead to a number of serious health and behavioral problems, including harsher parenting behaviors.[1-4]

> The parents of 8-month-old Ethan are running out of gas. While their first child learned to sleep on her own very easily, Ethan continues to wake multiple times per night. His mother used to breastfeed him back to sleep but this patterns is starting to take its toll on her, so now Dad will alternate in and give him some pumped milk. Both parents work outside the home, and their sleepiness is starting to affect their job, their mood, and their patience during the day. After the father nearly got into a car crash from momentarily falling asleep on the way home, he brings up the idea of letting Ethan "cry it out" rather than having one of them always assist him in getting back to sleep.

Parents of healthy 4- to 6-month-old infants are often told by their primary care doctor that their baby no longer physiologically needs to eat with such regularity. The subtle hint being conveyed here is that any continued fussiness at night begins to be less about hunger and more about the comfort and convenience of having a warm, loving, other person nestle you back to sleep. While some infants gradually become able to sleep on their own for long periods of time without parents needing to do much of anything special, around 30% to 50% don't,[5,6] and this is what leads to the extremely common dilemma of whether or not to be more directive in training an infant to be able to get to sleep and stay asleep without so much parental assistance. Of note, while the Holy Grail here is often referred to as "sleeping through the night," science tells us that all of us, young and old alike, typically wake up several times during the course of the night. The actual goal, then, is for an infant or toddler to be able to get to sleep and get *back* to sleep on her own.

## Sleep and Child Temperament

Over 40 years ago, the trait of rhythmicity was proposed as one of the nine core dimensions of temperament (see chapter 2 for more details) to describe how regular and predictable a child was with regard to eating, sleeping, and elimination habits.[7] These days, sleeping ability is not usually conceptualized as a temperament trait per se but could be considered as part of the broader family of child characteristics that vary between individuals and help define who they are. Sleeping characteristics do appear early in life and are under significant, but hardly complete, genetic influence[8-10] similar to more classic temperament traits like extraversion. All this suggests something that many parents already know, namely, that there are going to be both young children who struggle getting a good night sleep despite everyone's best efforts, and some who will sleep, well, "like babies," even as parents break every rule in the book.

It is also important to acknowledge that while this chapter will address the ways that child temperament can affect sleep, things can work in the other direction too, as anyone who has cared for an irritable sleep-deprived infant or toddler will readily attest.[11] A trait such as self-regulation or effortful control, for example, may be one of the first things to fly out the window among chronically tired children, not to mention their parents. Yet it is this same trait in a toddler that can be important in determining whether a parent's purposeful efforts to improve a child's sleep take 2 days or 2 months.

Thinking about our five temperament types, it seems logical to expect that at least three of them could require some adjustments to the default playbook when it comes to sleep training. From just a common-sense perspective (which can always be a little hazardous when it comes to behavioral science), we might expect that the general knowledge and recommendations about sleep training apply most closely to children in the moderate group, while those in the mellow group might be predicted to need little in the way of extra help to get through the night peacefully. The exuberance of the vigorous group, by contrast, might present as a little more of a challenge. With their higher levels of extraversion and surgency, these little guys might not want the party to end due to something as boring as bedtime. Consistency, and perhaps good old-fashioned resolve, might be at a premium for the parents of these children when it comes to sleep training. Those belonging to the agitated and anxious types, meanwhile, would likely also not be thrilled with the idea of going to sleep and staying asleep on their own, but here the key factor requiring attention is not the child's activity level but rather the degree of worry and fear that could be triggered by sleep training techniques. Indeed, the agitated group in particular could prove especially challenging due to the presence of high levels of *both* anxiety and activity.

> Three-year-old Joey gets anxious a lot. New places, new people, noises, and not being able to be close to his mother all get Joey riled up pretty quickly. Fortunately, Joey has always been a pretty good sleeper once he is able to fall asleep initially. As an infant, his mother would stay by the crib until Joey fell asleep. When Joey transitioned to a bed as a toddler, his mother tried to put together a consistent bedtime routine, which has helped him learn to fall asleep on his own. Lately, however, he has reported vague feelings of being scared and now often gets out of his bed at night to join his mother. With another baby on the way, Joey's mother very much wants her son to stay in his room and get to sleep after she kisses him goodnight.

The personality of the parents also deserve some consideration here. Most any parent is going to find techniques that push children to learn to fall asleep on their own to be somewhat stressful, but for those who fit the anxious or agitated type themselves, the level of parental distress may be particularly intense. Here, there may be a need to customize the approach by relying on additional support of a co-parent, if available, or by choosing a particular method that might be less likely to evoke a lot of crying from your infant or toddler. Other parents, by contrast, may be beyond ready to start these techniques yesterday. For you, the hazard might be in applying these methods *too severely*, which requires taking deliberate steps in the *other* direction. As described in chapter 3, it can be very useful to take stock of how your own traits play a role in each of these parenting topics so that you can be maximally aware of any potential biases that might arise in how you interpret scientific information and of the ways that your personality characteristics might require you to tweak your parenting approach to increase the chance of success.

By day, Michelle is a (mostly) delightful 2½-year-old-girl. By night, however, the family struggles mightily with her poor sleeping. Since infancy, Michelle has awoken multiple times a night. Michelle's mother has always felt uncomfortable with the idea of sleep training, but at the urging of their pediatrician, the parents began trying various methods to help Michelle settle back to sleep on her own. Not only did the parents find them extremely challenging and emotionally wrenching to do, they didn't seem to work. As a result, Michelle's parents gave up for a while, and the family settled into a routine in which a parent would lie down with Michelle until she fell asleep. This process often needed to be repeated at least once during the night. Since Michelle has been able to walk and have her own bed, the plan has changed to Michelle waking up and going into her parent's bed for the remainder of the night. After over 2 years of this routine, both parents are starting to find the long bedtime routines tedious, and they miss having a bed to themselves. As a result, the parents once again tried to employ some sleep training techniques, and once again they resulted in a lot of exasperation and tears on the part of both child and parents, but no improvement. In consulting with the pediatrician, she urges them to stay the course and persevere, warning them that Michelle might not learn to be as self-sufficient as she should be if the parents give in.

But before diving into how a child's or parent's traits might alter the approach to sleep training, we need to cover the basics with regard to these methods and tell the story about why the issue has engendered so much discussion and debate.

## The Controversy

Unlike other parenting dilemmas that will be covered in this book such as corporeal punishment and picky eating, the controversy is not really over the question of whether or not the techniques can *work* but rather over concern that the methods, particularly those that involve some component of an infant needing to "cry it out," result in psychological harm with regard to things like parent–child bonding, inner feelings of security and trust, and eventually the development of emotional-behavioral problems later in life. The camps on either side of this debate tend not to break down along purely political lines. In one corner are those who find behavioral sleep interventions to be safe and effective and generally a good thing for parents and children alike. The arguments from these folks supporting sleep training generally emphasize the effectiveness of these techniques, the negative consequences of poor sleep for both children and parents, the need for infants to begin developing self-soothing skills, and a lack of harm in enacting these methods.

Frequently these advocates tend to be more trusting of traditional Western-style medical practices, whose organizations such as the American Academy of Pediatrics and the American Academy of Sleep Medicine generally support using sleep training techniques. The latter maintains a website (www.sleepeducation.org) that offers information and advice on all things sleep related. When it comes to young children who don't sleep through the night, their message is clear. "There should be no reason for the child to get out of bed over and over again. You can take away things the child enjoys or create an awards system as an incentive." For infants, the advice is also unwavering: "Children should fall asleep in their own cribs or beds without being rocked to sleep. If a child must be rocked to sleep, then the child will not learn how to go to sleep without the parent's help."

In the other camp are those who find these sleep training techniques to be maladaptive at best and traumatic, even abusive, at worst. Some of the most vocal critics come from the attachment parenting perspective covered in the last chapter, which emphasizes the importance of empathy, attunement, and physical proximity between parent and infant to promote optimal development. The argument against sleep training includes the concern that such techniques harden parents from being emotionally attuned to their baby and essentially teach infants that expressing distress does no good because parents are not going to be there for you when you need them.[12] There are also often evolutionary arguments made that point out that mammalian babies are hardwired to call out when distressed and mammalian mommies are hardwired to respond to them.

As you might guess, the pro–sleep training camp generally is not as vocal or passionate about their position as the anti-camp, who see sleep training as a moral issue rather than a practical one. The exception to that, however, are the many critics of infant bed-sharing based on the link between it and sudden infant death syndrome (SIDS), a related topic that we will cover later in the chapter.

## What Is Sleep Training?

While taking thoughtful action to get infants and toddlers to sleep through the night seems like a very modern goal, the idea has been present for over a century. In 1906, one of the country's leading pediatricians, Emmett Holt, wrote in his book *The Care and Feeding of Children* the following about children who repeatedly awake crying at night.

> It should simply be allowed to "cry it out." This often requires an hour and, in extreme cases, two or three hours. A second struggle will seldom last more than ten or fifteen minutes, and a third will rarely be necessary. Such discipline should not be carried out unless one is sure as to the cause of the habitual crying.[13p164]

Ignoring the creepy reference to an infant as "it," the more modern term for this strategy is called *extinction* and is based on basic learning concepts of how behavior changes in response to rewards or lack thereof. In a nutshell, the idea is that an infant's crying at night is rewarded by the parent coming in and soothing her and therefore the crying behavior will persist until the parent stops giving the reward. More colloquially, this is the full monte "crying it out" approach that was described in the 1950s.[14]

Ironically, the famous Ferberization method that came onto the scene in the 1980s was initially designed to be a gentler version of extinction. In more scientific circles, this approach is referred to as *graduated extinction*, controlled crying, or even controlled comfort. Richard Ferber, then head of the Sleep Center at the esteemed Boston Children's Hospital, popularized this technique in his 1985 book, *Solve Your Child's Sleep Problems*,[15] although it is important to note both that others had been developing similar ideas[16] and that the graduated extinction method was not portrayed as a one-size-fits-all approach to all fussy sleepers. In the original edition, Ferber argued that his techniques were not only effective but that *not* using them could result in long-term impairment in a child's ability to regulate her own emotions, or self-soothe. He later backed off on this latter assertion due to a lack of scientific evidence.[17,18]

Despite the fact that the term *Ferberization* is virtually synonymous with the idea of a baby crying it out until exhaustion, Ferber has actually never advocated doing this. Rather, the graduated extinction method involves parents entering an infant's room and verbally trying to comfort "it," but doing so at progressively longer intervals. The details of the technique, like exactly how many minutes to wait before going back into the bedroom for a "check-in" on day 1 versus day 2, vary from study to study. Remember, these parameters are not being bestowed upon us on a stone tablet, and *people make this stuff up* before testing them in research studies. For those parents looking for a specific recipe to follow, Box 4.1 includes some detailed time suggestions for graduated extinction and other methods based upon a recent research trial.

---

### Box 4.1  Specific Instructions for Behavioral Sleep Interventions

---

#### Graduated Extinction/Controlled Comforting/Ferberization

1. Establish a consistent and warm bedtime routine.
2. Place the child in the crib/bed tired but awake and stay with the child until settled but still awake.
3. Say goodnight and leave the room.
4. If your child starts to cry or get upset, go the crib/bed and offer verbal comfort but do not pick up the child or turn on the lights.
5. For subsequent awakenings, increase the length of time before going into the room to offer brief comfort according to the following schedule.

| Night | 1st Delay (minutes) | 2nd Delay | 3rd Delay | 4th and Subsequent Delays |
|-------|------|------|------|------|
| 1st | 2 | 4 | 6 | 8 |
| 2nd | 3 | 5 | 7 | 10 |
| 3rd | 5 | 7 | 10 | 15 |
| 4th | 10 | 15 | 20 | 20 |
| 5th | 10 | 20 | 25 | 25 |
| 6th | 15 | 25 | 30 | 30 |
| 7th | 15 | 30 | 30 | 30 |

#### Camping Out or Chair Method

Begin with the usual calming bedtime procedure while making sure your child is tired, dry, and well fed. Then follow these guidelines.

1. Start at a baseline of you sitting or lying next to your child and assisting your child in getting to sleep with your touch and voice.
2. Once this routine is established, begin cutting back how much you touch, talk, and/or sing to your child until your baby can fall asleep without this extra help.

3. When your child is used to falling asleep without you needing to be too involved (this could be several days), move a little farther away from the bed/crib. You may need to talk or sing to your child at first but try not to do too much.

4. When your child can fall asleep with you a short distance away, move yourself even closer to the doorway and repeat. When successful with that, move out into the hall but still close by and continue the process until you are able to put your child to sleep and leave the room completely. *This could take a period of 1 to 3 weeks or more.*

5. If your child wakes overnight during the process, try to position yourself at the spot you were earlier in the evening. Stay there until your child goes back to sleep.

## Faded Bedtime

1. Pick a reasonable bedtime for your child.
2. Establish a consistent and warm bedtime routine.
3. If the child's sleep latency (time it takes to get to sleep) is more than 15 minutes, delay bedtime by 30 minutes the following night.
4. If the child's sleep latency is less than 15 minutes, advance bedtime by 30 minutes the following night.
5. Continue process until finding a time when latency is consistently less than 15 minutes.
6. Continue regular process of responding to infant awakenings during the night.

However, this is also one of those places where some customization is entirely possible based on the specific qualities of the child or parent. If you need to increase or decrease those intervals somewhat based upon your honest appraisal of your child or yourself, then do so. There isn't much science to argue that you *have* to wait exactly 2 minutes the first time your baby wakes up on day 1 and exactly 3 minutes on the second night.

A warning: before things get better, it is not uncommon for them to get worse as the child protests even more vigorously at the parent's absence. This phenomenon is called an *extinction burst*, and it is one of the main reasons that many parents who try the method have trouble seeing it all the way through. The good news is that this level of crying tends not to last very long, perhaps even just one (very tough) night. For those who may find themselves overly distressed at the idea of leaving the room of a crying infant, a variant of the technique called extinction *with parental presence* involves parents actually remaining in the room with the child but not actively trying to comfort her. This variant appears to work just as well as the standard version.[19]

## Beyond "Crying It Out"

While the term *sleep training* to most people equates with some use of extinction-based methods, there actually are a number of other behavioral treatments out there that may not have grabbed as many headlines but remain viable alternatives with solid backing from the published scientific literature. One of these techniques is called *camping out* or the *chair method*. Here, what gets varied is not time but *proximity* to the infant or young child. Starting at baseline during which a parent is generally right with the child and doing all of the work in getting her to sleep, the parent slowly does a little less while gradually moving farther away. From lying in the bed, for example, a mom might then try to sit in a chair next to the bed, and then move the chair farther away and even out into the hall, until she is not needed at all. This method can often take longer than extinction-based techniques but tends to avoid the difficult bouts of infants screaming at the top of their lungs.

Another procedure is called *faded bedtime,* which focuses a bit more on the initial getting to bed rather than later awakenings.[20] The idea is that a parent, while doing some enjoyable but calm activities together like reading a book, lets a young child stay up a bit longer until she is really sleepy on her own. Because of the increased sleepiness, the child falls to sleep pretty easily and without too much fuss. On successive nights, the parents then slowly creep this bedtime back little by little until they arrive at the magic hour when the child can consistently get to sleep fairly easily on her own. In a different version,[21] the parent puts the infant in the crib awake and sees how long it takes for her to fall asleep with a parent present. If it takes longer than 15 minutes, then the next night she goes to bed 30 minutes later. If it takes less, the infant goes to bed 30 minutes earlier. This procedure repeats until a bedtime is found that consistently results in a sleep "latency" of 15 minutes of less.

There is also a somewhat counterintuitive approach for middle of the night fussiness that actually involves waking an infant up *on purpose* (thus violating sacrosanct parental rule no. 1 of never waking a sleeping baby). In this plan, parents wake their sleeping child about 15 to 30 minutes before they estimate she would wake anyway on her own and do their usual routine of rocking or nursing. Under this plan, the groggy and disoriented infant will fall back asleep pretty quickly on her own and thus start learning how to fall asleep with minimal parental help (or intrusion in this case).

Finally, there exists a clever, if not a tad disingenuous, method called the *excuse me technique*, which can be tried for older toddlers and preschoolers who have more developed language skills. With this technique, the parent dutifully sits or lies down with the child at bedtime or during a nighttime awakening, pretending this night is going to be like any other in which the parent stays with the child until she falls asleep. This night, however, the parent makes up some excuse to leave the room briefly, like, "I just need to go to the bathroom" or "I need to go check on something downstairs." Generally, the child won't get upset over this minor interruption and will remain calm in bed. Over the course of the night or perhaps several nights, however, the parent lingers longer and longer away from the room with these lame excuses until at some point she just doesn't need to go in at all.

All of these methods are good alternatives to consider for parents who, based on their judgment of themselves or their particular child, might be hesitant to use techniques that include some measure of "crying it out." For example, the parents of a toddler who genuinely just doesn't seem to get tired at the expected time might be spared a lot of aggravation by using the faded bedtime procedure to find out what a more natural bedtime actually looks like, and then slowly moving it earlier if need be. Of course, all of these methods are generally bundled with the recommendation that bedtime routines be consistent, warm, and not overly stimulating and that babies, whenever possible, be put to bed while still awake so that they can begin to hone those important self-soothing skills. In addition, napping sometimes is recommended to be reduced somewhat when trying these techniques, although some children become more rather than less difficult to settle at night when overtired.

## Weighing the Research Evidence

### Co-Sleeping and SIDS

A related topic that needs to be discussed in the context of sleep training is the controversy about co-sleeping, particularly with younger infants. The American Academy of Pediatrics advises against co-sleeping with infants but recommends having infants in the same room as the parents. This, however, has nothing to do with the development of self-soothing skills or good sleep habits. Rather, it comes from research that has documented a link between co-sleeping and SIDS or the newer sudden unexplained infant death. The changing terminology is somewhat confusing and a more in-depth review can be found elsewhere.[22] For the purposes of this chapter, the issue at hand relates to what is known about co-sleeping and accidental suffocation.

These horrible tragedies are mercifully rare, but are still estimated to claim the lives of at least 2000 infants per year.[23] The rate of unintentional suffocation has also been increasing since the new millennium.[24] To date, the bulk of the scientific research continues to support the association between bed-sharing and SIDS with recent calculations indicating that bed-sharing raises the risk of SIDS almost threefold.[25] The reason the issue remains controversial is that the studies have been criticized for not adequately measuring and statistically controlling for other factors that may be the real drivers of this association, such as parental smoking and intoxication, or co-sleeping on riskier surfaces such as sofas.[23] When imperfect attempts to account for some of these other factors are undertaken, the risk of bed-sharing on its own tends to drop but often does not go away completely,[26] although in some studies it does.[27,28]

Another variable to factor into the equation is age. The research suggests that the risk associated with bed-sharing is highest for younger infants, like below 3 months of age,[25] compared to older infants. The American Academy of Pediatrics' 2016 report on the subject instructs parents to follow the "same room, different bed" policy for a year, but acknowledges that the co-sleeping risk is highest in infants up to 4 months of age.

Putting it all together, there remains continued evidence that bed-sharing is associated with an increased risk of infant death. The magnitude of this link is likely somewhat bloated because of other factors that are not always accounted for in these studies, but it remains difficult to dismiss away this association completely, as much as we might like to.

## Effectiveness of Sleep Training

Turning back to behavioral sleep training techniques for older infants, toddlers, and young children, the two primary issues that have occupied the minds of researchers in this area are (i) Do these techniques actually work? and (ii) Do they cause psychological harm over the short or long term?

Focusing primarily on the first question, noted sleep expert Jodi Mindell and some colleagues published an ambitious paper in 2006 that attempted to review all the literature to date on behavioral sleep techniques.[5] They were able to find 52 different studies that, combined, analyzed over 2500 infants and toddlers (average age about 20 months and about two-thirds were white). As best they could, they tried to classify the studies based on the type of technique(s) they used and the variables they measured to define success.

In total, an impressive 94% of the studies concluded that sleep training overall reduced bedtime resistance and night awakenings. Across studies, the percentage of youngsters who responded favorably to the intervention was 82%, although there was some variability around this number. Furthermore, improvement tended to occur quickly, often in a matter of just days. Furthermore, improvement tended to occur quickly, often in a matter of just days, and were found across different techniques (gradual extinction, faded bedtime, etc.), although graduated extinction and camping out were tested the most.

Aside from the sleeping benefits, many of the studies reported gains in other areas such as increased child security, decreased irritability, and improvements in a child's daytime behavior. For the parents, benefits were also found including reduced depression scores, increased sense of parenting effectiveness, improved marital satisfaction, and less fatigue. While few studies followed up their sample past 1 year, most of these benefits regarding sleeping and other factors were preserved at least in the short term.

Which technique was found to be *the best*? This good question is more difficult to answer, as most of these studies tested a particular approach against nothing. In addressing this issue, the Mindell paper concludes that "the direct comparison studies provide little evidence that one behavioral protocol is vastly superior to another,"[5p1269] although there was some evidence to support extinction techniques as working more quickly. This ambiguity is a bit of a mixed blessing. On the one hand, it would be nice for science to hand us *the answer* and declare one particular sleep training technique better than all the rest. On the other hand, the lack of a clear winner gives parents some science-backed flexibility for those who want to tailor the particular method they choose based on individual characteristics of the child or parent.

---

Ethan's parents decide to give sleep training a go and, after some discussion, decide to try a graduated extinction method in which they wait longer and longer before going back to comfort Ethan at night. They base this decision of their understanding of the science and an appreciation of everyone's personality. Ethan is not particularly anxious or active and seems to need about the expected amount of sleep as other infants his age. His parents, meanwhile, are emotionally prepared to take action and feel some urgency to change course as quickly as possible. The first night was rough as Ethan cried even louder when the parents did not immediately respond. Finally, however, he fell asleep. The parents continued with the program the next night. Ethan again resisted but fell asleep earlier than the first night. On the third night, Ethan awoke once and cried for 5 minutes before falling back to sleep on his own. Since then, his sleeping has improved dramatically with only occasional awakenings. The change has resulted in both parents feeling as though they have more energetic and positive interactions with Ethan during the day. They wonder why they waited so long to do this.

## Does Sleep Training Cause Harm?

Regardless of whether or not sleep training techniques work, parents also very much want to make sure that the methods don't have negative developmental consequences. Here, there is considerably less research, although more seems to be coming.

A handful of studies have tried to look at this question by following up as long as 6 years later on infants who did and did not receive sleep training during infancy. [21,29-31] These investigations have looked at a lot of domains including mental health and behavioral problems, quality of life, parent–child bonding and attachment, and levels of the stress hormone cortisol. The bottom line from these studies is that, over the long term, *kids who received sleep training as infants don't look any different than the ones who didn't.* Levels of behavior problems, rating of parent–child closeness, warmth and conflict, and scores related to the mother's level of anxiety, depression, and stress are all comparable. The authors of these studies have thus concluded that there is little evidence that behavioral sleep interventions result in long-term harm, and they hope that parents might feel more comfortable using sleep training methods to obtain the, albeit temporary, improvements that were found related to sleep and maternal mood.

## The Controversy Continues

These studies just described did get a fair amount of media attention and provided folks like pediatricians and other primary care physicians, as well as many parents, some needed scientific cover to counter the widely held position that sleep training works but results in psychological injury. For those already steadfast against sleep training, however, these studies did little to change their minds. Instead, the intensity of the sleep training debate heated up considerably to provide a counterpoint to all the publicity generated from these studies.

What ensued from the anti-sleep training camp were sharp rebukes of the research as being fatally flawed while offering in its place provocative references that supposedly demonstrated that sleep training instead resulted in significant and irrevocable brain damage. The language of some of these responses was powerful and convincing; that is, until one actually bothered to go to the reference section and actually look up the specific studies that were being cited. As an example, a blog post read by over a million people in *Psychology Today* laments that "over 2 million *Parents* readers have just been told that leaving babies to cry to the point of distress and beyond—to the point of potential neurological damage—has been proven safe and even that it's proper child-rearing."[32] The citation for this alarming claim about neurological damage, however, involves a study of monkeys who were given the stress hormone cortisol to drink for a month.

## It Depends

Sneaky tricks aside, the weight of the research evidence suggests that sleep training will be effective and well tolerated for the majority of infants, toddlers, and preschoolers. This statement does not mean, however, there aren't a number of places where the general recommendation or at least approach may need to be modified, based on the child's temperament and other factors. Despite impressive improvement rates for sleep training methods of 80% or more, there remains a significant minority of families still struggling. It can be tempting to dismiss these parents of "nonresponders" as simply *not doing it right*, but there likely are other factors related to the child's temperament and innate sleeping abilities that are at play. Thus, we now turn to how the overall science-based conclusions regarding sleep training might need to be adjusted a bit according to characteristics of both the child and the parents.

The need to fine-tune the general recommendations surrounding sleep training and its long-term effects has been well *acknowledged* by many child sleep experts, but this unfortunately has not translated into direct study. The 2006 review paper on sleep training by Mindell, which is still considered one of the definitive sources on the subject, states that "there are no systematic reports on patient or parent characteristics vis-à-vis the outcomes of the intervention." [5pp1271–1272] With the qualification, then, that we are starting to tread beyond what has been directly supported through scientific study and moving into areas of expert opinion, general consensus, and perhaps good old common sense, a case could certainly be made that some families might benefit from a slightly different approach or emphasis.

## Modifiers of Sleep Training Effectiveness

From a practical standpoint, it makes sense to divide the "it depends" discussion into factors that could modify the *effectiveness* of different sleep training methods versus those that might alter the psychological *impact* of sleep training on future development and well-being (see Box 4.1). Distinguishing the kids who simply need less sleep or who have more intrinsic sleep problems from those whose sleep problems are being driven by things like anxiety is not always easy. On the surface, the initial battles over sleep can look quite similar. The true nonsleepers, however, many of whom might belong to the vigorous temperament group, are more likely to manifest their nonsleeping behavior *everywhere*, regardless of setting or circumstances. In other words, they are just as active and restless in the parents' bed as they are in their own. These kids may also be more active during the day.

For these children, the standard extinction-based or camping out techniques could be much more of a struggle and could lead to increasing amounts of frustration, even resentment, on the part of the parents. A reasonable alternative here would be to emphasize other sleep-promoting recommendations, such as a predictable and calming bedtime routine every night. Limiting naps and late exposure to highly stimulating activities and screens might also be particularly important for this group of children. For toddlers and preschoolers, getting regular physical activity is always important, but it might be *really* important for these particular kids to discover the wonderful world of long walks or running laps around the house.

As mentioned previously, alternative sleep training methods such as bedtime fading could also be a good strategy to try sooner rather than later. In doing so, you may find out that a somewhat later bedtime is sufficient. While that realization could result in a little less "me time" at night, such a price is probably well worth paying compared to repeated nightly conflicts that only leave everyone feeling angry and ineffective.

Temperamentally anxious children are also likely to struggle more with traditional sleep training methods, especially those that involve extinction. In Ferber's 2006 book, he suggests some modifications of sleep training methods particularly for more anxious kids. These modifications included both the use of nonextinction techniques such as camping out (although he doesn't call it that) and providing for increased proximity of the parent.[15] In what many might consider to be a head-spinning contradiction to the Ferberization stereotype, he advocates for parents fully to sleep in a child's room, at least temporarily, when working with more severely anxious children. Only once the child's bedtime anxiety is diminished and the child feels more comfortable, an endpoint that could certainly take some time, does the parent then begin removing herself in slow gradual steps as the child gains mastery in falling and staying asleep on her own. Regardless of the specific temperamental traits that are being exhibited, the key may be for parents to approach a child's sleep problems inquisitively and flexibly as you reach for that extra cup of coffee.

> Joey's mother embarks on some steps to help Joey feel less anxious across many situations. She targets a few areas where she can supportively nudge Joey in taking small risks, like going into a swimming pool and spending a

little time at a friend's house, and then celebrates his successes. As Joey feels a greater sense of mastery, he gains some comfort in trying new things. After some time, Joey's mother begins a camping out technique at night, with full realization that this process will need to be taken slowly. They also adopt a cat from the local shelter who takes to Joey immediately. For a week, Joey's mother sits by the bed until Joey is completely asleep. Then she stations herself in the doorway while also strategically putting the cat's bed in Joey's room. She makes a point to talk to Joey from the doorway even though he can't see her as easily from his bed. When Joey seems comfortable and able to fall asleep with his mother in the doorway (this takes an entire month), she moves completely out to into the hallway. After another week, she is able to get Joey to stay in his bed as she moves about the entire apartment, at times making some noises on purpose to remind Joey she is still there. A week after that, Joey only seems to care about the cat being in the room with him.

## Modifiers of Sleep Training Impact

Aside from variability in sleep training effectiveness, there may also be particular groups of children for whom the negative impact of sleep training, in particular methods like extinction or graduated extinction, could be stronger. Obviously a better argument could be made here if there actually *were* some solid data that clearly demonstrated adverse developmental consequences as a result of sleep training, but science 101 teaches us that not proving the existence of something is not the same as proving its nonexistence. In the absence of more evidence, it certainly would seem to make sense to err on being cautious of things that even potentially could have detrimental effects.

Since the two issues of effectiveness and long-term impact will often be related (in that those children for whom sleep training methods are less effective are more likely to be exposed to them more intensely and for a longer period of time), we can expect that more anxious and agitated children might also experience more negative consequences of rigidly enforced sleep training methods. A couple nights of increased crying in the course of a graduated extinction program, for example, might be a small psychological price to pay for a temperamentally mellow infant, especially when considering the upside of having more energetic well-rested parents. By contrast, having ineffective extinction methods drag on week after week may be a different animal altogether for the infant or toddler who already struggles with significant anxiety.

The authors of an Australian study that followed groups of children who were and were not sleep trained up to age 6 admitted that they were not able to fine-tune their analyses on infants who were more anxious or had histories of abuse. Nevertheless, they speculated that "if supported by empirical investigation, there could be a case for using more gradual interventions such as adult fading instead of the more intensive graduated extinction."[31p650] Young children who have experienced trauma such as neglect often have learned from experience that a parent who departs may be truly unavailable to them no matter what happens. Consequently, their distress at being separated from a caring adult can take on a level of fearfulness that goes beyond what more securely attached children experience in a similar situation.

Lest some parents begin to worry here that using nonextinction methods inevitably means a trade-off in how well the techniques work, remember the, albeit limited, research that indicates that the various sleep training methods do not vary much with regard to their effectiveness. As such, a reasonable conclusion from all of these studies and expert opinion would be to start with methods such as camping out or faded bedtime for infants who fit into the anxious or agitated temperament type or who have other characteristics, like past trauma, that could magnify the impact of a parent not responding, even temporarily, to a child in distress.

A similar recommendation makes sense based on a *parent's* temperament or attitudes. Specifically, if the idea of using extinction techniques makes a mother or father nervous or uneasy, why not then try one of the other methods first? Camping out, faded bedtime, and other methods may take a little longer before one sees results, but this is probably preferable to a flood of guilt and the endless doubt of wondering if every behavioral challenge a child displays in the future developed because the parent didn't respond right away to a crying infant. Similarly, for those who might be inclined to feel guilty for *not* enacting sleep training methods and depriving the child the opportunity to self-soothe at night, remember that there is also no evidence that rushing to the crib whenever an infant starts to cry or co-sleeping with a toddler or preschooler results in any diminished ability for that child to regulate her emotions. As any parent will readily attest, there will be *plenty* of opportunities during the day to help teach and develop those important skills.

---

Michelle's parents decide to have a real talk about this. They would prefer if Michelle could get to sleep on her own at night and then stay in her bed until morning, but that just doesn't seem to be who she is. Moreover, these attempts are making Michelle's mother more and more uneasy about the whole process. Especially as the parents begin to realize that their daughter will not suffer a delay in her emotion regulation skills from a lack of sleep training, the couple concludes that, for them, these battles may be more trouble than they are worth. While they do find some success with the *excuse me* technique in getting Michelle to fall asleep better without a parent there, she continues to wake up and go into the parents bed more often than not. Rather than punish themselves, the parents decide to accept this as reality for at least the immediate future and look for more creative ways to find some romantic moments.

## The Bottom Line

Getting a good night's sleep is a very important function for both young children and their parents. For those kids who don't naturally fall asleep and stay asleep through the night on their own (which is most of them), a number of methods under the umbrella of sleep training techniques have been developed and tested in scientific studies. The take-home conclusions of this research is as follows:

- These methods generally work quite well.
- There are many techniques out there that don't involve children needing to cry alone for periods of time that also are effective.
- Research does not show that these methods result in psychological harm.
- Research also fails to demonstrate that *not* using sleep training techniques results in deficits in a child's ability to self-soothe.
- There remains evidence that co-sleeping with young infants can increase the risk of accidental suffocation.
- While not systematically studied well, there are reasons to suggest that some types of infants and young children would do better with methods that don't involve a measure of "crying it out."

All told, the research on sleep training indicates that really the only thing parents and young children stand to lose by *not* trying any type of method is, well, more sleep. That said, if comforting infants or co-sleeping with toddlers and preschoolers is really working just fine with all parties involved, science does not provide a compelling reason to suddenly change course.

I'm certainly not naïve or vain enough to think that this chapter will end the debate on sleep training while we await the results of more definitive scientific studies. Even those studies won't likely end the controversy, but hopefully now at least you can move forward more confidently with whatever decision you choose to make.

Good night.

## It Depends—Sleep Training

### General Summary

There are a number of different sleep training methods that research shows can be highly effective toward improving the sleep of both children and parents. These interventions have not been shown to have negative results on a child's emotional well-being.

| "It Depends" Factor | Adjustment |
| --- | --- |
| Anxious and agitated temperament type | Extinction-based techniques that involve some degree of "crying it out" may be less effective and not as well tolerated. Techniques such as camping out or faded bedtime may be preferable. |
| The vigorous type and general poor sleepers | Both extinction-based techniques and camping out may be less effective. Faded bedtime or other methods may be preferable. |

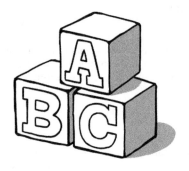

# 5

# Working

## Making Peace With the Childcare Wars

Any parent who has ever dropped off a screaming child at daycare, with a baby-sitter, or even at Grandma's knows that feeling. The wide eyes, the tears, the calls, the open arms—this is very tough stuff even for the most unflappable parent. You tell yourself that going to work will help the whole family and that your child will benefit from being around more kids his own age, but still that feeling in your gut persists as you force yourself to walk away.

Luckily, this pattern usually doesn't last for long. The next day often is hard but not quite as hard, and the day after that usually even better. Typically, by the end of the next week, it can be hard to give your child a goodbye kiss before he's off to join his new buddy at the playground. Still, the nagging thoughts continue. Have I traumatized my child? Am I missing out of the best part of parenthood? Am I being selfish for going to work and letting others care for my child at this young age?

> Larry and Hank have an adopted 3-year old boy named Xander. Both parents need to work to make ends meet, and so Xander spends most of the week at the most affordable childcare setting they can find close to home. But they've had some concerns about the quality of the care and at times felt that the level of supervision could be better. The teachers have expressed some of their own concerns about Xander and note that he has been more aggressive lately. Larry and Hank wonder how much of Xander's behavior may be due to the amount of out-of-home childcare he gets and if some sort of a change is needed.

Chapter illustrations drawn by Jaq Fagnant

*Parenting Made Complicated*. David C. Rettew, Oxford University Press (2021). © Oxford University Press.
DOI: 10.1093/oso/9780197550977.003.0005

It is easy to forget that many stay-at-home parents have their own repertoire of anxious questions swirling though their minds too. Will my child be more socially isolated at home? Will he not be ready for kindergarten? Can we afford the things we need? Is my sacrifice not to pursue a career going to make me bitter and resentful?

> Toni is a young single mother of a 2-year-old boy. She's overcome a lot but still struggles financially and, often, emotionally. She wants to be able to provide more for her son and knows she has the talents to succeed in the workplace, but she comes from a family where nonrelative childcare just wasn't something that was done. When the possibility of a good job arises, she thinks that this might be the moment to make a move but is hesitating because of the unknown impact this transition could have on her son.

One thing is for sure—both employed parents and those staying at home to raise their children are *working*. Reflecting on my own experience as a father and as a physician, I can tell you that an average day being the primary caretaker for my own kids (who honestly are not overly challenging) feels just about as strenuous as an average day of work. Certain tough days of seeing a lot of patients or being on-call is definitely more taxing than a typical day with the kids, but a more relaxing time at work with a few meetings, administrative duties, and teaching medical students and residents (who tend to be very well behaved) can actually feel like a break. Maybe that's just me—as certainly people are very different when it comes to what kinds of things feel more or less demanding.

For many parents, the need for early childcare is not optional. You may have to work to support your family whether you like it or not. But for others, in all fairness, the decision to use childcare providers versus raising young children at home really *is* at least partially a choice, which, of course, is why it can be so agonizing. One parent staying at home to care for the kids might mean a smaller house, less luxurious vacations, and a cheaper car, but that's a different ballpark than whether or not there is food on the table or a roof over your head.

Another aspect that can add pressure to the childcare dilemma is the need to make a decision early. Indeed, the reason that this chapter is in the first part of the book is that childcare arrangements often need to be made well before a child is born (some of you might even say *conceived*). Whether or not the consequences of nonparental childcare change when considering an infant versus a preschooler will be described later in the chapter. Regardless, however, the circumstances regarding childcare arrangements usually can't shift on a dime. Changing jobs, negotiating work hours, finding good childcare providers—all this takes considerable time and effort, which means that changing course when it comes to the family's childcare plans is not a decision to be made lightly.

Mia and Jeff both work in busy professional careers. Mia is an endocrinologist who works in a hospital clinic while Jeff works as a tax consultant. Financially, they are doing quite well. After the birth of their daughter, Katie, both parents returned to full-time work as Katie attended a well-regarded childcare center right on the hospital campus. Now 10 months old, Katie is showing some signs of being anxious and easily upset. Mia especially is now having second thoughts about the long hours away from her and feels the all too common bind of wanting to be a great parent while still having a rewarding career.

As more and more women in the 1980s and 1990s chose to pursue careers outside the home, often in addition to rather than instead of having children, questions quickly were raised about how this changing landscape affected children. The "day care wars" had begun,[1] with strong opinions being formed often along political lines that were usually well ahead of the scientific evidence. Those who challenged the status quo of stay-at-home mothers and hard-working but somewhat detached fathers risked being seen as subversive and "unnatural," while any critique of the growing movement of parents in the workplace and infants in childcare settings could be countered with accusations of supporting an oppressive system that accepted women only when they were "barefoot and pregnant."

The division between mothers who choose to forsake other careers to raise their young children at home and those trying to manage both employment and family life remains evident to this day. Maybe you're familiar with this picture: you're at a party or a community picnic or a school function, where you see the stay-at-home parents in one group and the employed parents in another. Resentment can build in both directions, fueled by political, religious, or cultural pressures, which can further harden parents' minds otherwise focused on simply trying to make the right call for themselves and their children. Much of this burden continues to fall disproportionately to women and mothers for a variety of reasons. Continued gender inequality with regard to pay, for example, puts additional pressure on women to leave their jobs when suitable and affordable childcare can't be found.

But can it be possible to step away from the rhetoric and look at what scientific information is actually known about young children who are raised in different settings? And does the magnitude of any differences that are found match the level of intensity that often accompanies this debate? To answer these questions, this chapter starts with what seems at first like a fairly easy and concrete question: whether nonparental childcare is better, worse, or the same compared to a parent raising a child at home. It will become evident quickly, however, that this seemingly simple question is anything but.

## Who's Taking Care of the Kids?

Nonparental childcare (most people who work in the industry prefer the term *childcare* to *daycare*) for young children is now the norm rather than the exception. According to the US Department of Labor, 60% of mothers with children under the age of 3 were in the workforce as of 2017.[2] At the turn of the new millennium, approximately 10 million children under the age of 5 were in nonparental childcare for at least 40 hours per week.[3] These statistics reflect a changing culture for women in the workplace and slow progress toward more egalitarian roles between men and women overall.[4] But given the assumption that parents are not going to make decisions that knowingly harm their children, the trends also suggest that the majority of parents see potential benefits of nonparental childcare for the entire family, including some directly for the child.

## Framing the Debate

### Potential Advantages of Childcare

The possibility of being able to get "the best of both worlds" by pursuing a gratifying career while also raising a family is a gleaming aspiration for many parents of any gender. Its attainment is thought to provide happier and more fulfilled mothers and fathers, but also a number of benefits for children, some of which occur directly and others that come along a more indirect route. Some of the major benefits include the following, which are also summarized in Table 5.1.

**Table 5.1** Claimed Advantages of Nonparental Childcare and Exclusive Parental Care

| Nonparental Childcare | Exclusive Parental Care |
| --- | --- |
| Child<br>• Increased socialization<br>• School readiness | Child<br>• Assured that caretaker really cares about the child<br>• Improved security and attachment |
| Parents<br>• Additional family income<br>• Satisfaction from career<br>• Needed break | Parents<br>• Joy of being so close to child<br>• Not feeling spread thin between competing interests |

1. *Increased socialization with other children.* Developmentally, it's important for children to interact with peers and nonparental care often provides a number of opportunities for young children to spend time with other similarly aged kids in a supervised setting. Of note, this feature would apply more for child-care centers than with other childcare situations like employing a nanny.
2. *School readiness.* Many kindergarten teachers will say that one of their most important tasks is to get children accustomed to the structure and routines of a school. Kids that have been in childcare are already used to an environ-ment that includes things like circle time, standing in lines, and working at a table or desk. Some centers also specifically teach early reading, writing, and math skills, which could increase confidence and enthusiasm for early academics in elementary school.
3. *Additional income.* Clearly, one of the driving forces for the number of children in daycare and early childhood education programs is economic. Even after all the expenses of daycare are subtracted, a second income can make the difference between just getting by and being able to afford things that can enrich a child's environment.
4. *Parental peace of mind.* It's common to hear from adults who spend a lot of time in the company of young children that they really can come to crave adult company and interaction. After the 10th back-to-back game of Chutes and Ladders, even partisan bickering on cable news starts to sound appealing. This understandable need for grown-up contact can also put a burden on the parent working outside the home who then becomes the caregiver's sole lifeline to the outside world of adults. Of course, many adults also gain a great deal of satisfaction and fulfillment from doing meaningful work that can be hard to get from other sources.

## Potential Advantages of Parental Care

From the other perspective, the parent who delays or gives up another career to be home with her child often does so with the belief that no one can better care for her son or daughter than she can and that staying home gives that child the sense of security and consistency she so richly deserves. The personal reward, apart from any inherent benefit to the child, is that the parent is there to be a part of everything—each little milestone and achievement. When baby takes her first steps, you are there. When baby says her first words, you are there. Overall, the joy that comes from playing and loving a child, and being able to watch her de-velop, is yours every single day.

It also may be true that the fervent pursuit of getting the best of both worlds when it comes to having a career and raising a family can sometimes leave you feeling like you got neither world. It certainly is not uncommon to hear mothers and fathers say that they feel like bad parents when they're working and bad workers when they're parenting. Finding that famous work–life balance can prove to be extremely challenging to pull off, especially as demands change on either side. Better, some might argue, to focus on one thing or another, at least until a child is old enough to go to school.

Then, of course, there are the reports that have been surfacing for decades that daycare can result in some problems down the road. In the years preceding the onset of the daycare wars, a strong scientific literature was building that showed how important a child's early environment was for future behavior and functioning. Studies on attachment, the bond created between an infant and parent that provides a foundation for emotional stability and trust, created a compelling backdrop that argued strongly for the importance of loving, sensitive, and responsive parenting. In this context, it was not surprising during the daycare wars to see claims that optimal child development requires the continuous caregiving of a single person.[5,6] In 1986, psychologist Jay Belsky wrote a controversial paper entitled "Infant Day Care: A Cause for Concern?"[7] opining that children who spent too much of their early months in daycare might develop to be more aggressive and disobedient than those cared for at home. The study caused a considerable negative reaction and prompted accusations that Belsky was misogynistic and antiquated in his views.[8] As the childcare wars began to heat up, one of the few places of general agreement was the need for more high-quality research on this topic.

## The Big Study

One of the sources of all the controversy over childcare was that the whole topic turned out to be much more complex than many people originally thought. Parents were looking to the science to give them an overall thumbs up or down, but it quickly became clear that many other factors needed to be considered and, further, that it was some of these other variables that were making the available research at the time so inconsistent and easy to cherry-pick for advocates on both sides of the issue. The *quality* of nonparental childcare, for example, might be an important factor, especially relative to the quality of the home environment. Also potentially relevant might be the *exact quantity of time* a child received nonparental childcare at *particular stages* of development. The exact *type* of nonparental childcare (centers, relative-care, nannies, etc.) might also figure into the mix. Then, of course, there is the other side of the equation to consider, namely what to use as the outcome measure. Should it be a child's academic or cognitive ability, levels of behavior problems, quality of attachment to the parents, or some combination of them all? And, of course, all this still left the possibility of the answer being, "It depends," based on the particular characteristics of the children themselves.

Sorting out all of this would be a tall order. Fortunately, however, the scientific community recognized this complexity and made a decidedly bold response. Indeed, what sets the debate over nonparental childcare apart from every single other parenting controversy covered in this book is the fact that, in this case, the US government directly set out to settle the issue by designing and implementing a mother-of-all massive study that could hopefully lay the question to rest. That effort was the National Institute of Child Health and Human Development (NICHD) Study of Early Child Care and Youth Development, which will be referred to as the NICHD study going forward. While it began way back in 1991, it remains one of the largest and most comprehensive studies ever done on the subject.[9] This huge 100+-million-dollar project followed for many years over 1300 children and their families from 10 geographical areas. It was designed specifically to overcome many of the methodological shortcomings of earlier investigations. The NICHD study's primary objective was "to examine how variations in nonmaternal care are related to children's social-emotional adjustment, cognitive and linguistic development, and physical growth and health."[10p4] Those reading closely might have just noticed the word *nonmaternal* rather than *nonparental*, and, yes, the study did not count care by the mother and the father as equivalent, something that today would have probably led to a major protest by Baby Bjorn–wearing stroller-pushing fathers everywhere (with my support!).

Politics aside, the researchers focused on two main questions: (i) How do children who were exclusively raised at home by their mothers (defined as less than 5 hours per week of regular nonmaternal childcare) compare to those who received nonmaternal childcare? and (ii) How differences in the type, quality, or amount of nonmaternal childcare children received before kindergarten relate to various child outcomes?[11] This commitment to rigorously look at childcare *quality* both in and outside the home represented one of the most important advances of this study that was often missing from previous research. By "outcomes," the investigators meant repeatedly measuring a number of different domains including cognitive and language skills, attachment security, school readiness, social competence, and levels of behavioral problems. Data were collected initially every 3 to 4 months beginning in infancy and became more widely spaced out up until the final official Phase IV of the study as the children began high school.

It is important to note that families were *not* randomized for this study. Rather, the researchers assessed the childcare that the parents had chosen for their kids. This is important because the extent of parental versus nonparental childcare tends to be associated with *other* factors that also could be related to a child's adjustment and development, as the researchers indeed found. For example, mothers who exclusively cared for their young children also tended to have less education and more depressive symptoms than mothers who utilized childcare.[10] If maternal depression and education matter in a child's development, then it might mistakenly appear that exclusive maternal care is the variable of interest when in fact it is these other variables. The researchers did their best to measure and statistically account for these other factors, but doing so results in more complexity and the need to deal with a lot of moving and mutually interacting parts.

## What the NICHD Study Found

Now let's look at some of the major findings of the study from the hundreds of journal articles that were published from these data.

### Parenting Still Matters

Interestingly, one important conclusion about this study of nonmaternal childcare was the importance of, drum roll please, *parenting*! As the researchers write, "the primary conclusion is that parenting matters much more than does (nonmaternal) child care, so parents might make decisions that allow them to have quality time with their children."[11p113] The importance of good parenting also held regardless of whether or not the child spent time in regular childcare. In other words, the impact of parenting when it came to things like child cognition, social abilities, language, and levels of problem behaviors doesn't get watered down for those kids who also got a chunk of their childcare from others. By good parenting, the study is referring to qualities described as *authoritative* in chapter 3—things like being warm and supportive while still setting reasonable limits. It also refers to an absence of harsh and overly critical behavior like yelling, name calling, and, of course, any kind of abuse.

### "Exclusive" Parent-Raising: No Better or Worse

As for one the study's primary stated goals, another important finding was that comparisons between children who were exclusively raised at home yielded no differences on any of the major outcome domains than those children who received at least some routine nonmaternal childcare. Keep in mind here, however, that "exclusive" childcare by mother could include up to 5 hours per week of nonmaternal care. It is also important to note that this comparison lumps together a kid getting 6 hours of nonmaternal childcare per week and a kid who gets 46.

## The Importance of Quality

For those kids who did receive nonmaternal childcare, another big takeaway from this study was that childcare *quality* was a key factor overall. By quality, the researchers took into their overall calculations statistics like the adult-to-child ratio, worker training, and average group size as well as more "process" characteristics related to the individual childcare providers like being sensitive and responsive, providing a stimulating but not overwhelming environment, and being involved and enthusiastic without being intrusive. The size of these associations between childcare quality and various outcome measures was moderate and, as mentioned, not as large as the impact of parenting. Nevertheless, across the many ages studied, higher-quality childcare was associated especially with improved achievement on cognitive and language domains but was also present with regard to areas like child behavior and peer relations.

## Hours of Childcare and Behavioral Problems

Quantity of daycare was less related to various cognitive and language outcomes, but there were some areas where it was important. Specifically, there was evidence that, after controlling for other variables, the overall amount of hours spent in childcare was associated with incrementally more behavioral problems at age 36 and 54 months,[12] although it has been pointed out that some of this association was probably due to longer hours in poorer-quality care.[13] In one analysis, the rate of elevated levels of "externalizing" problems, things like being defiant or aggressive, was 5% for children who had received less than 10 hours per week of nonmaternal care up to age 4½ but16% for kids who typically received 30 hours per week or more.[1] This discrepancy continued as children entered kindergarten as shown in Figure 5.1.[14]

In terms of there being a stronger effect of care hours spent during one period of time versus another (e.g., infancy versus preschool years), no consistent result was found, and overall "it is the cumulative quantity of nonmaternal childcare . . . that is most predictive of socioemotional adjustment rather than the amount of time in nonmaternal childcare during any particular period."[12pp999-1000]

## Childcare Setting and Development

The setting for nonmaternal care—the child's home, another person's private house, or a big childcare center—did not have a major impact on child outcomes once quality and quantity of care were taken into account. That said, there were small but statistically significant associations between children spending proportionately more time in a daycare center and some both positive and negative outcomes across a child's first 5 years. Specifically, more time in childcare centers

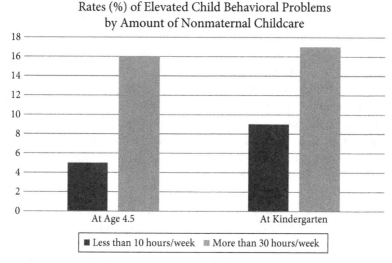

Figure 5.1 Increased percentages of children with elevated rates of behavioral problems prior to and during kindergarten among children with full-time nonmaternal childcare (more than 30 hours/week) compared to minimal nonmaternal childcare (less than 10 hours/week).[1,14]

tended to be associated with kids doing a little better cognitively with regard to things like language skills and memory but a little worse behaviorally (more disobedience and aggression), although not to a level that would cause concern in doctors and other professionals.[15]

## Do Children in Daycare End Up Securely Attached to Their Mothers?

Of particular interest to many parents and researchers alike was whether or not nonparental care affects the important attachment bond between child and parent. By the time the NICHD study began, there had been some research documenting that children who had experienced longer hours of daycare as infants were more likely to be deemed insecurely attached to their mothers. In particular, they were more likely to display the "insecure avoidant" pattern in which a child shows less interest and concern with a mother being present or absent with the child than would be expected.[16] The NICHD study found that, broadly viewed, spending time in daycare and other forms of nonparental care was unrelated to whether or not a child was rated as securely attached at around

15 months of age and that, predictably, what instead mattered was how sensitive and responsive the mother was. Looking at the raw percentages, a total of 61% of infants cared for at home by their mother were rated as securely attached compared to 70% among those going to a daycare center. This difference was not found to be statistically significant. More fine-tuned analyses, however, did reveal that the combination of lower maternal sensitivity/responsiveness *and* either lower-quality childcare or high number of hours of care was related to the likelihood of being insecurely attached. The study also showed that specifically boys who attended more than 30 hours per week of center-based care were more likely to be rated as insecurely attached at age 15 months.[17] This finding, however, didn't persist as the children got older.

## Takeaways from the NICHD Study

In total, this large-scale study makes a strong case that, when it comes to children receiving early nonmaternal care from nannies, other relatives, or daycare centers, the quality and characteristics of that care *matter*. This conclusion is very much a double-edged sword. On the one hand, parents can be reassured from the findings that high-quality childcare did not appear to be harmful to children and, in fact, seemed to put some children at an advantage, especially when it came to academics. However, the same results bode much less well for the large number of children receiving poorer-quality care. In the NICHD study, which provided at least a snapshot of what average nonparental childcare looks like across the country, the overall conclusion was that only about 9% of kids were receiving an ideal amount of positive caregiving with the majority of young kids getting "some" or a "fair amount."[18] For most parents, the idea of their young child receiving "some" positive caregiving while they are at work is not going to cut the mustard.

Similarly unsettling was the link between increased quantity of time in childcare settings and increased rates of child behavioral problems and child–adult conflict. In the final commentary from a published book on the NICHD study, noted childcare expert Sharon Ramey stated that when it comes to some of the thorny associations found between the quantity of nonmaternal care and negative outcomes, "no one seems to like hearing about these findings. Everyone wants to find the flaws in the study and its measures, because this would be much easier than confronting the call-to-action findings."[10p433] By *call to action*, she refers to the data on both the amount of "unacceptably low-quality" care and the findings related to more hours of childcare being related to increased amounts of some behavioral problems and levels of child–adult conflict.

## Childcare Impacts Later in Life

When the children in the study were about 8 years of age, most were assessed again to see if some of the previous associations were able to withstand the test of time.[10] These studies found that some of the earlier effects were still present while others appeared to fade away. The kids who had experienced higher-quality child care prior to kindergarten, for example, continued to do better in academic areas such as math, vocabulary, and memory. In addition, the children who spent more time at center-type childcare settings continued to show the mixed-bag effect of higher memory abilities but more difficult relationships with both teachers and mothers. Other associations, however, such as the relations between higher amounts of daycare and problem behaviors, no longer held. Interestingly, some new associations were also found at this time period, including a link between more hours in nonmaternal care, lower social functioning, and poorer study habits.

When children were in the sixth grade, early childcare quality remained associated with higher vocabulary scores, while more hours in center-based care was associated with higher levels of rule-breaking and aggressive behavior as rated by teachers.[3] A new link was also found in that children who had experienced *increasing* nonmaternal childcare from 3 to 54 months tended to have lower vocabulary scores.

While the study is now officially over, a few attempts to follow this group have continued, with the participants as of 2020 being around 18 years old. One report looking at these children into adolescence found that many of the major findings endured with regard to quality of early care being related to improved cognitive/academic achievement. More difficult to interpret was an association found between quantity of early nonparental care and higher levels of risk-taking and impulsivity at age 15.[19]

## No Surrender

After all this, one might have reasonably predicted and hoped that a mega-study like this one would have finally brought peace, or at least clarity, to the daycare wars. To some degree it has: the position that childcare overall is some toxic force on society has become increasingly difficult to support on scientific grounds. At the same time, however, the very comprehensiveness of the study also became its Achilles' heel. With so many analyses of so many measures of so many outcomes (and at multiple time points), there were inevitably going to be some inconsistencies in the data that require interpretation, synthesis, and, yes, human judgment. This, then, can very quickly lead to the potential for politicizing, cherry-picking, bias, and ultimately conflict even between the scientists directly involved in the study. This is exactly what happened. Jay Belsky, a psychologist and researcher with the study, was particularly embroiled in controversy (again) when he suggested publicly that some of his colleagues were whitewashing over some of the more troubling associations with full-time childcare to make women feel less guilty about going to work. In turn, he was criticized for grandstanding to the press, being overly alarmist in his claims, and generally not getting along well with others in the research team.[20] Since the study's official end, different pieces of this study continue to be deployed by writers trying to make the case for[21] *and* against[22] daycare. While this trend will certainly continue, you are now equipped with a much more balanced understanding of this crucial study and many of its important but frustrating details.

## Yes, Other Researchers Have Looked at Childcare Too

This chapter has given a lot, perhaps too much, attention to the NICHD study. There are good reasons to do so, but certainly the research on the effects of nonparental childcare doesn't begin and end with this single investigation.

Fortunately, some of the other more recent major efforts have reached similar conclusions. One such study in the United Kingdom called the Effective Provision of Pre-School Education project found results similar to those of the NICHD study, although it focused on nonparental childcare that occurred during the preschool years rather than the entire time between birth and kindergarten.[23] Another important paper was a meta-analysis in 2010 covering 69 individual studies that looked at mothers who worked outside the home. This study also found that overall there was little association between maternal employment and child cognition or behavior, but with more nuanced results to be addressed soon.[24] An even more recent study that garnered some significant media attention also found that daughters of mothers who worked outside the home were more likely to be employed themselves as adults and earn more money while sons, on the other hand, grew up to spend more time with family activities.[25]

## It Depends

The NICHD study and others like it go a long way to help people understand how unproductive it is to lump all nonparental childcare into one big box that is either good or bad. How good the care is certainly matters, as does in some instances the amount and type of childcare. These efforts also very clearly demonstrate that, even for kids who receive a lot of nonparental childcare, other factors such as parenting, socioeconomic status, genetics, and many others figure heavily in determining a child's overall development.

> For Larry and Hank, there may not be much choice in whether or not they work outside the home and so they decide to focus on the overall quality of care Xander is receiving. With less supervision, lower levels of positive interactions, and larger child-to-adult ratios, Xander's more irritable temperament is not getting redirected. Larry and Hank do some searching for other childcare settings (a nice guide that can help evaluate childcare providers is the Positive Caregiving Checklist that can be downloaded from one of the summary brochures of the NICHD study).[26] With some effort, they find one. It is a bit more expensive, but they decide it is worth the investment and make a change.

In addition to the main factors already described like overall quality and quantity of care, are there other variables that need to be considered that can modify or alter the impact of nonparental care on children? This is where we turn next. In the process, we'll bring back some of the case examples to illustrate how all these swirling things to consider can converge into specific recommendations for specific families.

## Does Gender Really Matter?

While most studies do not find major gender differences when it comes to the effects of nonparental childcare, some studies have suggested that boys may be slightly more negatively affected by lower-quality care or longer hours of care.[13,18] Overall, however, a child's sex or gender did not significantly change the general conclusions made about the effects of daycare on child development.

## Economic Disadvantage

There is evidence that high-quality childcare and early education programs are especially beneficial to children from economically disadvantaged backgrounds.[27-29] The previously mentioned meta-analysis of maternal employment showed a particularly striking pattern with maternal employment being associated with better outcomes for children with single parents or with families using welfare assistance but with some negative outcomes for middle- and upper-class families, especially when the child was very young while mothers worked. High-quality daycare has also been shown to help reduce aggressive and oppositional behavior among children from lower-income households.[18] Of course, it is the same economically disadvantaged families that are less likely (at least in countries like the United States) to be able to obtain high-quality nonparental childcare, and it is this mismatch that has generated some of the political campaigns to push governments to support universal access to high-quality affordable childcare.

With more information in hand, Toni has a tough decision to make: she feels uncomfortable leaving her son with strangers and wonders if this uneasiness will eat away at her should she return to employment. On the other hand, a strong childcare center could improve her son's ability to do well at school, and this resource could leave Toni more available to advance in her young career and improve their economic status. The key for Toni will be finding a high-quality childcare center that she can afford that will also give her peace of mind during the workday. Fortunately, for Toni, there's a new state program that might partially subsidize the cost of a nearby childcare center that gets great reviews. Overall, she thinks this could be a good decision for herself and her son.

## Should Babies Be in Childcare?

Recall that much of the concern raised about developmental effects of daycare in the 1980s was directed especially at infants who received extensive nonparental childcare in the first months of life.[16] Since then, studies looking at whether infant childcare was related to insecure attachment have been quite inconsistent. The NICHD study offered some insight into this confusion by showing the need to take into account other factors. Specifically, the researchers did not find evidence that, by itself, the age at when children received nonparental care had a major effect on a child's emotional or cognitive status later on. It did, however, find that the early childcare *combined* with other factors, such as a mother being less sensitive in her care, did predict toddlers and preschoolers being less securely attached. Others studies that have focused directly on child behavior and levels of problems like aggression or rule-breaking have found that they can be associated with longer hours of infant nonparental care, but these links can fade with age.[1,30] The 2010 meta-analysis also found that maternal employment that occurred during a child's first year of life was slightly related to lower child achievement scores (IQ and academic testing) whereas employment that occurred in the child's second or third year was related to slightly *higher* achievement scores.

All this leaves us in a bit of an unsettled place when it comes to decisions about infant childcare. While parents can be comforted by data showing that working full-time when a child is an infant does not lead to sad and emotionally fragile kids, there may be some circumstances when early and extensive infant childcare is not ideal. Such a conclusion, which is supported by many but certainly not all research studies, may be disquieting to some but can result in a balanced and cohesive strategy for parents who have options for their childcare situation.

## Child Temperament

Theoretically, there are lots of ways you could think a child's temperament might impact the response to nonparental childcare. It would certainly seem logical, for example, to expect that more social and extraverted children might enjoy the stimulation of big daycare centers while more anxious or shy kids could find this same environment stressful. On the other hand, one could also argue that over the longer term the daycare centers are helpful for less extraverted kids because it helps them overcome their fears and prepares them for the school setting.[31] Similarly, we could imagine that more temperamentally challenging kids tax even very devoted and loving parents.[13] In these cases, a tag-team approach that involves a nanny or a childcare provider might help all caregivers maintain enough gas in their tank.

The NICHD study measured child temperament, under the idea that this was an important factor but, surprisingly, didn't find that it really changed their overall conclusions that much. This may, however, have resulted from their use of an older and, some might argue, outdated temperament scale. More recent re-analyses, however, have found that the link between higher quality of childcare, lower levels of behavior problems, and better social skills when children were 4 to 5 years old seemed to hold only for kids whose temperament was rated as more "difficult" in infancy (akin to the agitated type described in chapter 2).[32] Furthermore, a relook at the sample when they were in sixth grade revealed that the association between higher-quality early childcare, lower levels of behavioral problems and child–teacher conflict, and higher reading ability was also present only for children with more difficult temperaments.[33] Altogether, this had led some to put forth the idea that children with more challenging temperaments are more susceptible, for better *and* for worse, to the quality of their daycare environment, just as they are to better and worse parenting.[33,34] Such a view really expands the idea of what it means to be a "sensitive" child.

Some other studies that have measured temperament differently, using the framework described in chapter 2, have also found some intriguing findings. In a couple interesting studies of young children who were enrolled in full-day center-based childcare, researchers found that some of these children experienced rising levels of the stress hormone cortisol as the day progressed if they were in childcare but had decreasing levels of cortisol if at home. This pattern was especially true for kids rated as higher in traits of shyness and negative emotionality and lower in effortful control.[35,36] In her review of this research, well-known temperament researcher Susan Crockenberg concluded that temperamentally fearful children show greater stress responses to full-time, center-based childcare, especially in lower-quality childcare settings.[13,36] One complication of these cortisol studies, however, is it is difficult to know whether a child's increase in cortisol levels at a daycare center reflects true stress versus just higher levels of arousal and engagement.[37]

Then there are the studies indicating that nonparental childcare might actually help more sensitive infants and toddlers be less anxious over time. One study looking at the stability of temperament from infancy to toddlerhood did find that more emotionally reactive infants showed less behavioral inhibition (fearfulness and reticence with new people and situations) as toddlers if they had received nonparental childcare.[38] A subsequent study did not find an impact of childcare on anxiety stability for older children, but quality of care was not measured.[39]

How do we square these conflicting lines of research? The answer might be in looking at how different studies dealt with the number of hours kids spent in nonparental childcare. Specifically, the studies suggesting possible negative effects of childcare on temperamentally vulnerable children tended to look at kids who were getting a lot of nonparental care while studies showing a positive effect set the bar at lower threshold, such as 10 hours per week. Putting this together, it suggests that there may be a bell-shaped curve here when it comes to the optimal amount of daycare for more anxious and socially reticent children. A moderate amount might be helpful in getting kids exposed to more social situations, a required step to overcoming anxiety, while too many hours may get to be overwhelming.

For Mia and Jeff, there may be some signs that the current childcare situation isn't ideal for their daughter Katie, who is looking as though she is somewhat anxious temperamentally. The 40-plus hours of childcare per week may be experienced by Katie as simply too much. Furthermore, there is less evidence that nonparental childcare will exert much of an academic edge to this child who already is the recipient of a lot of socioeconomic advantages. Mia is also starting to feel somewhat uneasy about the childcare arrangements—a factor deserving of attention itself. Changing their busy and fulfilling work lives, however, is no small task. After a lot of challenging discussions with both themselves and their employers, the parents work out an arrangement in which Jeff will cut back his hours in the summer and fall while Mia will decrease her work hours in the winter and spring tax seasons. When Katie is a little older, they will reassess this plan.

## The Bottom Line

Does nonparental childcare early in life have a positive or negative impact on development relative to at-home parental child-rearing? This seemingly straightforward question got complicated fast as we began considering all the different characteristics of the daycare, home environment, and the individual child. Even a large, well-designed, and well-funded study built specifically to settle the subject struggled to provide easy answers, although much has certainly been learned. Clearly, the sum of the evidence does provide a strong message that high-quality daycare is not something to be feared by parents. Children who spend time being cared for by relatives or nannies or in childcare centers develop their cognitive, social, and emotional abilities similarly to children who are cared for primarily by their parents. Furthermore, parents do not lose their influence on a child's development just because other people are participating in their upbringing.

But beyond these broad and, for parents working outside the home, comforting conclusions, the scientific evidence also does contain some important caveats:

- Higher-quality nonparental care (if you can find and afford it) can bestow some advantages for children both academically and behaviorally, particularly for those who come from disadvantaged backgrounds.
- Similarly, poorer-quality care can lead to more negative outcomes with more temperamentally challenging kids showing the most sensitivity to the quality of the nonparental care.
- There still is a lot of controversy and inconsistency about the link between the *amount* of nonparental care (and when in a child's life it occurs) and child behavior. In several studies, modestly higher levels of some behavioral problems like defiance and aggression have been associated with increased hours in childcare settings, particularly when there are concerns about parenting quality at home.
- More center-based childcare was modestly related to some increases in child cognitive variables but also some increases in negative behaviors.

- Long daycare hours might be especially stressful for more anxious kids, although not all studies show this to be the case. At the same time, some anxious children might benefit from a moderate amount of nonparental care as a way to help them learn to be comfortable with new people and new situations. That "sweet spot" with regard to the exact number of daycare hours will be different for different kids.

In trying to put all these findings into perspective, it looks like there could be some grounds for peace in the long-fought daycare wars. Indeed, one could argue that what has been so polarizing to many people isn't necessarily the science itself but the proposed solutions to those findings. Take, for example, the opinion that extensive hours in especially lower-quality childcare settings is suboptimal for many children. What makes this position controversial isn't that the opinion is not scientifically grounded but that society's general response to it has been that it is the *moms* who need to sacrifice their careers to fix the problem. If solutions instead were sought through remedies such as (i) trying to improve the quality of daycare, (ii) advocating that maternal and paternal leave policies be more supportive of parents trying to maximize time with their newborn without penalty, and (iii) the expectation that fathers step up their childcare responsibilities for kids who might benefit from fewer daycare hours, it seems likely that a much broader consensus could be built.

## What About You?

Finally, while you're immersed in considering what's best for your child, remember that it is okay to consider how various parenting choices would affect *you*. Would staying at home with the kids simplify family life and lead to feelings of satisfaction, or would it breed regret and resentment? Would having a nanny that your child loves feel like a relief or a threat? There are many studies at this point demonstrating that the mental health of the parents influences the mental health of their children for better and for worse. This implies that mothers and fathers who feel fulfilled, engaged, and accomplished will be able to transmit those positive qualities through their parenting to their baby or toddler, regardless of whether those good feelings come from their career, their time at home with their child, or any combination of both.

## It Depends—Nonparental Childcare

### General Summary

Child development is more strongly related to the qualities of the home environment regardless of whether or not the child receives nonparental childcare. Overall, few differences are observed between young children raised exclusively by a parent at home and those who have other childcare arrangements.

| "It Depends" Factor | Adjustment |
| --- | --- |
| Daycare quality | Higher-quality nonparental childcare is associated with higher cognitive and academic abilities and better behavior. |
| Daycare quantity | Long hours of nonparental childcare is associated at some ages with higher levels of behavioral problems and child–adult conflict. |
| Socioeconomically disadvantaged backgrounds | Improvements related to high-quality nonparental childcare may be particularly true for children from more disadvantaged backgrounds. |
| Aggressive children/agitated type | These children may be more susceptible to the benefits of both high quality nonparental care and the negative effects of lower-quality care. |
| Anxious type | These children may do best with a medium amount of nonparental childcare that allows them to overcome their fears without becoming overwhelmed. |

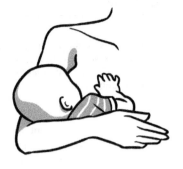

# 6

# Got Milk?

## The Case for Breastfeeding Leading to Smarter and Happier Kids

The inclusion of breastfeeding as a parental "controversy" might surprise some people. It's benefits, after all, are extremely well established, right?

Well, yes and no. It is true that breastfeeding is associated with lower rates of a number of health problems, ranging from respiratory and ear infections to things like allergic disease, asthma, diabetes, leukemia, and even sudden infant death syndrome. These benefits have been found across a large number of studies, and while the link between some of these conditions and breastfeeding may still be debated in some circles, there's strong scientific consensus that, overall, breastfeeding is a valuable practice that offers some real advantages for your baby's health.

That said, many proponents of breastfeeding also include as benefits various cognitive, developmental, and behavioral dimensions such as improved bonding and attachment, lower levels of behavioral problems, and higher intelligence. Here, the science becomes a bit murkier and deserving of a closer look to see if the level of evidence matches the level of advocacy, especially as breastfeeding increasingly becomes viewed not only a medical imperative but a moral one.

The culture surrounding breastfeeding has taken a number of twists of turns in modern history.[1] The universal practice of breastfeeding began to be challenged in the Victorian age as wealthy mothers used wet nurses to provide for their offspring. With the introduction of formula in the 1950s, breastfeeding began to be viewed by the rich and poor alike as antiquated and no longer necessary,

Chapter illustrations drawn by Jaq Fagnant

*Parenting Made Complicated.* David C. Rettew, Oxford University Press (2021). © Oxford University Press.
DOI: 10.1093/oso/9780197550977.003.0006

causing rates in the United States to plummet, especially as larger numbers of women joined the workforce. The pendulum then began swinging back again in the 1970s as scientific research began to describe the medical benefits of breastfeeding and as families began to push back against what was viewed as a world increasingly detached from its natural roots. As government and medical groups began actively promoting breastfeeding and discouraging formula, the cultural pressure, especially in white middle- and upper-class circles where parenting was developing into a competitive sport, began to mount. As it did, mothers who weren't able to breastfeed or who simply choose not to started to feel judged and scorned. Today, online accounts frequently document the harsh criticism that follows non-breastfeeding mothers who get blamed for selfishly choosing personal convenience over their baby's needs in the face of what is perceived as overwhelming evidence that infants must be breastfed except under extreme circumstances.

This level of scrutiny and moral righteousness surrounding breastfeeding even now has a name, *lactivism*, as described in the popular 2015 book.[2] In response, there has been mounting an ever more vigorous and visible defense that argues not against breastfeeding per se but rather what is seen as an out-of-proportion fervor that has outstripped the science and morphed breastfeeding into an unjustified yardstick by which to measure good versus bad mommies. A subtext behind these discussions also relates to race and class, especially as breastfeeding has undergone such a huge reversal in its association with socioeconomic status. A hundred years ago, breastfeeding was very much the practice of lower-income families. Today, it is just the opposite.

Chloe is expecting her first baby. Like many soon-to-be moms, she is excited but also quite nervous about the road ahead. Chloe has not had an easy life. She struggled in school but, with a lot of perseverance, was able to obtain a high school diploma. Growing up, money was always very tight in the family, and her parents often had to rely of government assistance to get by. Soon after graduation, Chloe started working at a fast-food restaurant where she met a man whom she thought might be someone she could marry. Unfortunately, this man ended the relationship after he found out Chloe was pregnant. Chloe is now back living with her parents. Her obstetrician talked with her about the benefits of breastfeeding, but Chloe's own mother isn't convinced that it is "worth the fuss."

In this crossfire of mixed messages, we plunge into the politically charged world of breastfeeding and the evidence that links it to improved developmental and behavioral outcomes. The goal of this chapter is to look more deeply at the science in a way that allows new and expecting parents to be truly informed about the existing research on whether breastfeeding is causally related to happier, smarter, and more well-adjusted children.

## The Official Position

Let's start with some basics. According to the Centers for Disease Control and Prevention, approximately 83% of new mothers in the United States initiate breastfeeding, although there are some significant cultural and socioeconomic differences embedded in this overall number, with breastfeeding rates higher among older, higher income, and white and Latina women compared to lower income, younger, and African American women.[3] Across a baby's first year of life, breastfeeding rates tend to fall to around 58% at 6 months and to 36% at 1 year.

These higher but still modest rates of breastfeeding occur despite quite unambiguous advice from expert health organizations. The official recommendation from both the World Health Organization and the American Academy of Pediatrics in their most recent 2012 guidelines are for exclusive breastfeeding (i.e., no other foods or liquids) for an infant's first 6 months of life and then continued breastfeeding with complementary foods for 1 year or longer, as shown in Table 6.1.[4]

This guidance is based on reviews of the medical literature by organizations such as Evidence-Based Practice Centers of the Agency for Healthcare Research and Quality that conclude, fairly strongly, that there is compelling scientific evidence that breastfeeding is causally associated with a wide range of positive health outcomes. Fueling some of the intensity surrounding the advocacy of breastfeeding, a 2010 study in the prominent journal *Pediatrics* calculated that

**Table 6.1**  Official Breastfeeding Recommendations

| | |
|---|---|
| American Academy of Pediatrics | Unless specifically not recommended for medical reasons, exclusive breastfeeding for an infant's first 6 months of life followed by continued breastfeeding for up to 1 year or longer as complimentary foods are introduced |
| World Health Organization | Unless specifically not recommended for medical reasons, exclusive breastfeeding for an infant's first 6 months of life followed by continued breastfeeding for up to 2 years or longer as complimentary foods are introduced |

From the American Academy of Pediatrics.[4]

the United States would save the lives of over 900 children per year, in addition to 13 billion dollars, if the rate of breastfeeding at the 6-month-old time period rose to 90%.[5] Another recent study from Brazil, where breastfeeding is less related to social class, showed that breastfed children had an income that was 20% above the average.[6]

When it comes to more specific effects of breastfeeding on development, behavior, and intelligence, however, the language of the American Academy of Pediatrics' recommendations on breastfeeding starts to soften and hedge a bit. The authors of the report cite studies that support the conclusion that breastfeeding leads to more intelligent and well-adjusted children but acknowledge that these "outcomes are confounded by differences in parental education, intelligence, home environment, and socioeconomic status."[4pe830] This qualification sounds like a fairly technical detail that can and should be ignored, but in fact a huge chunk of the case for breastfeeding rises or falls on the interpretation of that phrase. More on that soon.

## Why the Science of Breastfeeding Is So Annoyingly Debatable

At the risk of too much self-promotion, I'll contend that the debate over breastfeeding and improved child cognition and behavior is a wonderful example of why books like this are needed. Indeed, it is fair to say that the debate over the developmental effects of breastfeeding, perhaps more than any of the other parenting controversies covered in this book, is less about the *absence* or underappreciation of the scientific data and more about the degree to which the science that exists is really good enough to be trusted. When people go to the trouble of trying to figure that out, the conclusions that are reached on this question run the gamut from the view of breastfeeding as one of the most critical elements there is for a child's positive development to the view that, at least when it comes to things like behavior and intelligence, breastfeeding itself is a nonfactor. If you are an agnostic but concerned parent trying to make the best decision for your baby, it can feel like watching a tennis match as your head swivels to read the opinions coming from the two perspectives. How is it possible, you might very legitimately ask, that smart people with good intentions look at the same body of research and wind up concluding such vastly different things?

A big part of the answer to that question, as was discussed in chapter 1, lies within the complex psychology behind how we wind up believing the things we do and the remarkable ways that a sincerely motivated quest for objective truth gets twisted and sidetracked by all kinds of subtle biases coming at us from different directions. This is a fascinating study in and of itself, but it is not the focus of this book to try to understand why you, me, or your favorite radio talk show host struggles so mightily in being able to perceive and interpret information like Major Spock rather than Captain Kirk.

Another large source of confusion, however, comes not from our own frequencies of psychological interference but from the science itself. As awesome as it would be to have the ability to separate parenting hype from nonsense without having to deal with dry and laborious things like statistics and research study design, it simply isn't possible. To understand what science actually knows about a particular topic, and particularly to understand how things get so messy in the process of figuring that out, you have to wade into the weeds a bit and spend a little more time than what is required to read a headline or a tweet.

Parents are often prepared for the science about topics like love and happiness to be a bit muddled, but on the surface it seems like we should have questions regarding the benefits of breastfeeding wrapped up by now. After all, breastfeeding is a fairly clear and concrete thing to observe and measure. Intelligence is too, with all of our validated instruments that have been around for decades. A study could just measure IQ in a large group of children and then compare the numbers between those kids who were breastfed as infants to those who were not. What's the problem?

This analysis actually has been done many times over, and the outcome consistently shows that breastfed children do tend to score better on intelligence and behavioral dimensions later in life.[7] The reason, however, that such an approach doesn't end the debate is because mothers are not flipping a coin and being randomized to breastfeed or not. Instead, mothers make their own choices when it comes to breastfeeding, and the studies are simply following along. Scientifically, that wouldn't be a big problem if the decision to breastfeed or not was a pretty random one and not based on a bunch of other factors, but it's not. Rather, women who choose to breastfeed, at least in Western societies, tend to be somewhat more educated, have higher incomes, and make healthier decisions with regard to things like smoking, drinking, and eating. Some studies also show that women who breastfeed tend to have (on average, of course) slightly higher intelligence themselves.[8] Because of these things, a simple comparison of the intelligence or behavior of breastfed versus non-breastfed kids can't tell us whether it was really the breastfeeding itself that caused these gains or whether it's these other factors that are really driving the difference, as breastfeeding tags along for the ride. IQ is known to have a fairly strong genetic influence, for example. That means if women with higher IQs also tend to be more likely to breastfeed, then what looks like a causal effect of breastfeeding might actually just be a boring old inheritance of a parent's cognitive abilities.

When it comes to the skeptics who believe that the hand regarding breastfeeding's role in cognitive and behavioral development has been vastly overplayed, this tends to be their number one complaint of the existing science. Sure, they argue, you can find plenty of studies that document an association between breastfeeding and intelligence, but most of them have not measured and taken into account all these other variables that we know are important. Furthermore, they maintain, those relatively few studies that actually do control for things like the mother's IQ tend to have much less impressive results, as we will see.

Meanwhile, many advocates of breastfeeding who maintain that it really does have direct benefits on child behavior and intelligence also come prepared with legitimate criticisms of the existing research studies. They just tend to point out *different* flaws and focus their criticism on studies that *don't* find evidence that breastfeeding makes a difference. One problem that is often highlighted has to do with how breastfeeding is measured. Specifically, they take issue with the practice of some studies to create a single yes/no breastfeeding variable that lumps together the infant that was breastfed sporadically for 1 month and the infant that was breastfed exclusively for 10 months. If what matters more is the duration or exclusivity of breastfeeding, then such lumping can seriously jeopardize a study's chances of finding any positive result. As a researcher, you might try to avoid altogether making that tricky call of how much breastfeeding should be considered *enough* and instead declare the duration of breastfeeding your main variable of interest. That's great, but what if the relation between breastfeeding and intelligence isn't a nice linear pattern? If it turns out that there is more of a threshold effect when it comes to breastfeeding, with important benefits up to some point but then less incremental value after that, such a pattern would be easy to miss unless someone was specifically looking for it. Then there is that thorny problem, which is really one of the fundamental premises of this book, that the effect might not be the same for all children. It might be possible, for example, that an infant born into a supportive and stimulating environment with two intelligent parents might not gain that much *additional* benefit from breastfeeding while another child born to poor parents with less intellectual endowment themselves could reap a much larger reward with breastfeeding. Or it could be just the opposite.

---

Sandy and Richard are trying to do everything right for their new 2-month-old infant girl. The couple met when they were both in medical school, and now both of them have settled into busy but more manageable schedules. When Sandy finishes her maternity leave, a full-time nanny will be joining them at home. Sandy has worked hard to breastfeed her new daughter, but it has not come nearly as easily or as naturally as she had expected. Several times she has experienced clogged ducts, which have been painful and difficult. She is starting to consider a switch to formula, but both she and Richard are worried that doing so will cause her baby to be less intelligent and less attached to them than she otherwise would be.

We are left, then, with the arduous but probably more fruitful task of having to wade through the studies that analyze what mothers choose to do naturally when it comes to breastfeeding while trying to keep all of these other complicating or confounding factors at bay. Unfortunately, given the fact that all studies possess some methodological *flaws,* there are always grounds for someone to dismiss pretty much any scientific finding that one would rather not believe. The question for this chapter is whether or not there are broader patterns or signals in the data that are strong enough to rise above the shortcomings of each individual study so that a more substantive case for breastfeeding as a cause for better child behavior and intelligence can be made.

## The Link Between Breastfeeding and Child Intelligence

Studies on breastfeeding and child development are plentiful, so much so that there have been several attempts to summarize them through meta-analyses, which, if you remember, is a method of combining data from multiple studies into a single overall study to arrive at a more global conclusion. One of the first groups to try this in 1999 concluded, on the basis of combining 20 previous studies, that breastfeeding was indeed associated with an increase in child IQ of about 5 points, which actually was probably more like 3 points once you factored in the effect of these other variables such as maternal education and socioeconomic status.[9] Another meta-analysis in 2007 found again that breastfeeding was associated with improved cognitive ability later in life but noted that many of these studies may not have sufficiently controlled for these other confounding factors.[10] Overall, this was the overall theme of the research being done with studies generally showing significant associations between more breastfeeding and better cognitive abilities but with the magnitude of these effects being more modest (in the 2 to 5 IQ point range with perhaps additional benefit for babies born prematurely) once other factors are taken into account.[9,11] For years, studies looking at IQ and cognitive abilities were much more common than those looking at child behavior and attachment.

So far so good. Breastfeeding advocates had their scientific evidence while needing to acknowledge that maybe the strength of the effect is not as big as originally thought. But things didn't end there, and over the past 10 to 15 years, newer studies have come out that have ironically increased the controversy rather than diminished it. In 2005, a group of researchers from Scotland pointed out that there were very few studies on breastfeeding and child intelligence that took into account maternal intelligence and that this was really weird given the fact that everybody knows that intelligence has a fairly strong genetic influence. To remedy that, they looked at the role of maternal intelligence in their sample of over 12,000 children in the United States while also going back and summarizing older studies that controlled for maternal IQ. What they found for their own data was that the effect on intelligence for breastfeeding not only was reduced but essentially went to zero. Then they found the same result when grouping together the relatively small number of studies that controlled for maternal IQ in addition to other potential complicating factors.[8] They noted, however, that the studies looked at different groups of people and the ones that found a preserved association between child intelligence and breastfeeding even after controlling for maternal IQ were done with samples that tended to have a higher proportion of lower income and disadvantaged families.[12]

The public message from this study, as well as some others like it, was that variables such as maternal intelligence and parental education were the true driving factors behind *all* of the apparent link between breastfeeding and intelligence, not just some of it. At this point, the scientific battle lines were drawn. In addition, many parents who had increasingly felt criticized and shamed for not breastfeeding saw some vindication in these research findings, while advocates for breastfeeding started to become concerned that studies like this would erode some of their long-standing efforts to improve breastfeeding rates in the United States and beyond.

The dueling studies and ensuing coverage in the media has continued. A 2017 study looking at a large Irish sample used a new kind of statistical analysis that is supposed to make observational studies look more like a randomized trial.[13] In doing so, they found no significant link between breastfeeding and either cognitive ability or behavioral problems at age 3 or 5 with the exception of a very small decrease in hyperactivity scores at age 3 only. Another recent study, however, did find a link between breastfeeding duration and specifically verbal IQ.[14] This study did not control for maternal IQ per se but did include maternal educational and income, which are strongly related. Interestingly, a study designed to look also at soy formula found small but significant gains in early cognitive tests relating to breastfeeding, with little difference in the type of formula preparation.[15]

A methodologically strong study published in 2013, which did control for maternal IQ (and other things like level of cognitive stimulation and emotional support in the child's home), also showed a persistent association between IQ and duration of breastfeeding.[16] The authors calculated that, controlling for other factors, each month of breastfeeding was associated with an additional 0.35 points on verbal IQ and 0.29 for nonverbal IQ when children were tested at age 7, translating into about 4 points for a year of breastfeeding. In trying to explain how this study continued to show links with breastfeeding while similar studies that also controlled for maternal IQ and home environment did not,[12,17,18] the authors point to their examination of breastfeeding *duration* as the critical variable rather than a more global yes/no approach.

The most recent summary and meta-analysis on observational studies of breastfeeding and intelligence found an overall bump of 2.6 to 3.4 IQ points, depending on whether or not the study controlled for maternal IQ.[19] When the authors focused on what they considered to be the very best and most rigorous studies, the difference was still there but fell to just under 2 points.

## The PROBIT Study

As the debate over breastfeeding has intensified, so has the call to researchers to come up with study design that could do a better job of evaluating actual causality between breastfeeding and child development. Obviously, an actual randomized trial would be ideal here from a purely scientific point of view, but how many moms are going to give up their choice to breastfeed or not based on some random assignment? Even if some would, the ethics of such a study would definitely come into question.

One study, however, did find a clever way around this problem. The Promotion of Breastfeeding Intervention Trial (PROBIT) followed over 17,000 mothers and their children from Belarus, a country with fairly low breastfeeding rates.[20] Rather than creating randomized groups who either breastfed or not, they instead introduced a program designed to augment and support breastfeeding and administered it to *half* of the study sample. This resulted in there being two groups: moms who did what they were going to do anyway and moms who received extra incentives and support to breastfeed as much as possible. The program produced its desired scientific effect with the two groups being equivalent in lots of other variables that might feasibly also affect breastfeeding rates (things like maternal education and age and numbers of other children at home). The promotion of breastfeeding also worked well with mothers in the "experimental" group tending to having breastfeeding rates that were higher than the control group when infants were 3, 6, 9, and 12 months of age. Even bigger differences (43% vs. 6%) were found in the rates of exclusive breastfeeding when infants were 3 months old.

Intelligence testing conducted when the children were 6 years old showed that the breastfed kids had a verbal IQ which was a whopping 7.5 points higher than those in the control group, while the group differences for performance (nonverbal abilities) and overall IQ were not statistically significant despite being relative large. This verbal IQ difference was impressive, especially when considering that many of the mothers in the control group also breastfed. In raw numbers, the full scale IQ of children in the control group was 101.9 (with 100 considered average) compared to 109.7 in the breastfeeding augmented group (a 110 score would be considered above-average intelligence).

Depending on the analysis, there was also some indication that teacher ratings of academic performance were slightly higher in the breastfeeding promotion group for reading and writing. The study concluded that there was considerable support for an effect of breastfeeding, particularly with regard to verbal abilities, but noted that the exact magnitude of these differences might be a little off due to some methodological problems that they encountered. The study also looked at many different types of behavior including hyperactivity, aggression, and relationship quality with the parents, and, here, no advantages related to breastfeeding were found.[21]

The difference in verbal IQ, especially using this randomized design, certainly made some waves but was not without its critics. One problem that was officially pointed out by some of the authors of studies that have not found effects of breastfeeding on behavior and cognition was that the people who rated intelligence in the PROBIT study knew the status (control vs. experimental group) of the children they assessed and thus may have been biased in their ratings.[22] The authors of the PROBIT study anticipated this flaw and so had the intelligence of a smaller number of children evaluated by raters who did not know if the child was in the augmented breastfeeding group or not. In that subgroup, the verbal IQ difference dropped to 2.8 points and no longer was statistically significant. All told, this "definitive" study becomes a little less definitive, unfortunately.

Another type of study design that has been employed to improve the confidence in making any conclusions about breastfeeding involves comparing siblings in the same family in which one child was breastfed and the other was not. Since both children have the same mother, many of the other factors that might also relate to child behavior and intelligence are held constant.

One of the previously mentioned studies by Der, Batty and Deary illustrates quite convincingly how what looks like a breastfeeding effect can slowly melt away as one looks more closely.[8] Studying over 3000 American mothers and their children (preterm babies excluded) over many years, the researchers measured not only breastfeeding but a number of other potential factors that might impact a child's IQ. They also conducted a separate comparison between families in which the same mother breastfed one infant but not the other or when siblings were breastfed for different durations. Before doing all the fancy controls, children who were breastfed were found to have an IQ of between 4 and 5 point higher than the ones who were not. Once maternal IQ is thrown into the mix, however, the association with breastfeeding drops by over 70%. Add in other variables like maternal education, poverty, and age, and the IQ advantage falls to less than a point and is no longer statistically significant, although there was some evidence that the association was not linear with cognitive benefits of breastfeeding evident (even controlling for other factors) only among those who were breastfed for more than 6 months. The comparison of siblings, furthermore, found no differences in IQ based on breastfeeding status (yes or no) or duration, as did another study that used a similar type of approach.[12] These studies also found no effect on other behavioral measures such as levels of hyperactivity or parent–child attachment.

A third study of adolescent sibling comparison, however, did find differences in cognitive ability.[23] An interesting side note for this study and possibly an emerging theme that is coming to light is that this study oversampled low-income families. Like some other studies described here, the authors first looked at the associations with breastfeeding and a number of outcomes without controlling for potential confounding variables or focusing on siblings within the same family. As expected, breastfeeding was positively associated with lots of things, from reduced medical problems to child–mother closeness to even grade point average. And, as expected, most of these differences disappeared when comparing siblings who have been breastfed different amounts. However, scores on a vocabulary test remained significantly related to breastfeeding duration. The authors of the study concluded boldly that "this study provides the strongest nonexperimental evidence to date that having been breastfed improves cognitive ability."[23p1797] While the study was criticized for relying on a teen's memory to say if and how long he was breastfed, the authors did find that their cognitive variable remained significant even when breastfeeding was coded as yes or no, which most adolescents presumably would know.

## How Might Breastfeeding Change the Brain?

One of the reasons that many people believe the research that supports the developmental advantages of breastfeeding is because biologically it makes sense. Breastmilk contains a lot of nutrients, most notably long chain polyunsaturated fatty acids such as docosahexaeonic acid (better known as DHA) and arachidonic acid, which have been shown to be important in the growth and development of nerve cells as well as in the signaling from one neuron to another.[24,25] Infancy is a period of rapid brain growth and organization, and there is evidence from both human and primate studies that is beginning to connect the dots between breastfeeding, maternal diet, and offspring cognitive abilities.[14,26–29]

While some of this evidence comes from animal studies, others are done with actual humans using brain magnetic resonance imaging (MRI) scans. These studies can be hard to pull off for technical reasons (such as infants continuing to squirm around in MRI scans no matter how many times you tell them to keep still), but some studies conducted with older children are starting to emerge. One of them was done by child psychiatrist Joan Luby and colleagues at Washington University in St. Louis, Missouri.[30] What makes this study relatively unique was that they had information about breastfeeding, IQ, *and* the brain. With this trifecta, they found not only that breastfeeding was associated with increased IQ but that this link could be explained *through* the breastfed children having more grey matter brain volume in some subcortical regions (areas deep inside the brain).

Another theory about how breastfeeding might enhance development is, at least on the surface, noticeably less technical, and focuses on the stimulation and increased skin to skin contact. This close interaction then helps build a sense of security, which, in turn, facilitates behavioral and cognitive growth going forward. It has been shown in mice that the amount of licking and grooming a mouse mother does with her pups (this is the mouse equivalent of good parenting) is associated with better neurodevelopment.[31] While there is not much debate about the positive impact that early nurturing experiences have on children, the question here relates to how much *more* bonding occurs with breastfeeding compared to bottle feeding, as many parents (including a lot of dads) are quick to note that bottle feeding is hardly some robotic process and can also be a very intimate and warm experience for both baby and parent. A possible way to tease out any effects of breastfeeding from the effects of breastmilk would be to compare direct breastfeeding to infants who are often given expressed breastmilk in a bottle, but to my knowledge this unfortunately has not been done.

## A Summary of the Research

At this point, it probably is more than evident why a definitive and final verdict on this important topic has been hard to come by, especially one that fits into a single sentence or two. In full disclosure, I should say that I had hoped that the case for breastfeeding as a strong causal agent in improving behavior and cognition would be a slam dunk. All three of my own kids were breastfed, and while I can take no credit for that as a father, it would have been heartening to see all of that effort reflected in science that overwhelmingly demonstrates how important breastfeeding was for their emotional-behavioral development.

The research, however, tells us that it is not a slam dunk. When it comes to things like reduced levels of behavior problems, better social relationships, or a heightened sense of security, the studies are fairly consistent in showing that any associations found relating to breastfeeding status can be explained by other factors such as the home environment, socioeconomic status, and other qualities of the parents that tend to be more common among breastfeeding mothers. This should certainly not be interpreted to mean that non-breastfeeding moms lack other positive characteristics or come only from lower-income or education backgrounds. These conclusions, rather, come from relatively small *average* differences in child behavior between large groups, with there being lots of exceptions to the rule. Nevertheless, these studies overall fail to show that breastfeeding has a direct causal effect on these behavioral dimensions after accounting for other relevant influences.

By contrast, the story for child cognitive abilities and intelligence is a little different. While it is true that what initially looked like rather sizeable gains in IQ from breastfeeding appear to be overinflated, there continues to be evidence for there being a smaller effect, in the 2 to 3 IQ points ballpark. Certainly, not all studies show this, but amidst all the conflicting results, there does emerge some reasons to have confidence that breastfeeding can indeed result in these modest increases in cognitive ability. First, many studies converge in showing cognitive improvement particularly for *verbal abilities*—something that is not easily explained by chance or those pesky confounding factors. Second, those increases in verbal IQ are there for arguably the most definitive study we have at this point, namely the PROBIT study, which used an experimental design. Third, more recent reviews and meta-analyses continue to find a preserved association between IQ and breastfeeding even after controlling for maternal IQ and other important variables. And, fourth, the neuroscience research is beginning to demonstrate *how* this association might be occurring with regard to brain development.

A 2 to 3 IQ point bump may not sound like a huge difference to some people, but it is not something to take lightly (I certainly wouldn't want to hand over 2 to 3 IQ points without a fight). Remember also that this is an average, which means that there are some children for whom the effect is minimal to nonexistent and others where it can be much larger. This, then, brings us to the important question of what we actually know about possible "it depends" factors when it comes to the developmental benefits for breastfeeding. If the effect is not the same for every child, does the research give us any clues as to which children are likely to benefit the most from breastfeeding and for whom any advocacy efforts might be more specifically targeted?

## It Depends

Unlike some other kinds of "parenting behaviors," breastfeeding has not been shown to have a differential impact based on a child's temperament, although honestly people really haven't looked that hard to find out. Consequently, we'll need to look at other domains where the positive effects of breastfeeding may be most prominent.

## Maternal Diet

As might be expected, there are some preliminary indications that the beneficial effects of breastfeeding are strongest among mothers who have the healthiest diet.[14,32] This research has focused most, as previously mentioned, on the intake of those healthy polyunsaturated fatty acids found in things like cold-water fish. As it is likely that many of these same mothers had a similar diet *before* the baby was born, it can be a little complicated teasing out the effect of a good diet prenatally and a good diet during breastfeeding.

## Babies Born Prematurely

Another group that might stand to benefit even more from breastfeeding are babies who are born prematurely. Unfortunately, some of the big studies discussed here excluded premature infants in their research. Luckily, others have specifically focused on them. A more recent study done just with premature infants did show IQ gains associated with breastfeeding, although unfortunately maternal IQ was not controlled for in the analyses.[32]

## Parental Education and Intelligence

Perhaps the most important "it depends" factor could be summed up as follows. *The positive developmental effects of breastfeeding may be strongest among the mothers who are statistically the least likely to do it.* How's that for a public health challenge? Certainly the IQ and cognitive benefits were found in studies who included mothers across a broad range of educational, intelligence, and income levels,[33] but there is a signal that some of the strongest results are found when looking at mothers from more disadvantaged backgrounds. Recall that the PROBIT study was conducted in Belarus and not some wealthy American suburb. In the Der study that generally argues against breastfeeding effects on intelligence, the authors also notice the relation between the average socioeconomic status of the group being studied and the likelihood that the study finds a significant association between breastfeeding and higher IQ.[8] While admittedly a politically more sensitive issue, the same principle may similarly apply to parental IQ, meaning that infants of parents with lower IQs may stand to benefit relatively more from the effects of breastfeeding than infants of high IQ parents. Indeed, just as I was writing this chapter and coming up with this idea (I swear), a paper came out supporting the hypothesis that the cognitive benefits of breastfeeding might be strongest, on the order of two to three times as strong, among children with a lower IQ.[34] Other studies have not looked at their data this way, *but they could*, and perhaps this new study (and this chapter, of course) will inspire some researchers to go back and check.

Putting this all together, the idea is that the infant born to really smart and highly educated parents who are able to provide everything they can think of to create an enriched environment for their baby might be reaping relatively less cognitive benefit from breastfeeding, even though this is the kind of family most likely to do it. Conversely, the infant from a more disadvantaged family born to parents with less intellectual abilities could well be the one who stands to gain the most.

Sandy and Richard dig deeper to learn more about the link between breastfeeding and child development. In taking an objective look at their own situation, they see that their daughter is fortunate to have a lot of advantages that improve her chances of being a bright and emotionally healthy child with further breastfeeding probably not adding that much to the equation. While Sandy isn't sure yet if she wants to stop trying, she feels much less guilty about the prospect of not breastfeeding for the full year and is better able to concentrate on providing a warm and nurturing environment for her young infant.

## Public Health Implications

In the course of promoting these conclusions about breastfeeding, my hope is certainly not to provoke scorn and judgement on mothers who don't and especially can't breastfeed, but rather to help stimulate more thinking about how we, as a society, can remove some of the extra obstacles disadvantaged families often face when trying to breastfeed their new baby.

Chloe talks to her well-informed obstetrician who listens to her concerns and then provides education about the benefits of breastfeeding. She explains to her that not only could her baby be protected from many medical problems as a result of her breastfeeding but that there's evidence that babies born into more disadvantaged environments like hers might reap a proportionately larger reward when it comes to cognitive gains. Chloe remarks that it is about time that her hardships lead to an advantage in *something*, and the two get to work discussing how they can make her breastfeeding attempt most successful and what kinds of supports she will need.

It seems really challenging to be able to deliver a truly science-informed message about the behavioral and intellectual advantages of breastfeeding without sounding like a killjoy, a boring professor, or a complete snob. Public health messages need to be both inspiring and simple—like, *smoking is really bad for you*. Indeed, there's an argument to be made that the less dramatic and more nuanced arguments for breastfeeding are better left to scientific conferences than public health campaigns. Right now, the dominant message the public hears when it comes to breastfeeding is neither subtle nor qualified— basically, women who can breastfeed should do so for as long as they can. Much of the vigor in these recommendations come from the many medical benefits of breastfeeding that are outside the domains of behavior and intelligence where the scientific evidence is not so messy. The problem is that these benefits aren't as inspirational to mothers who might be somewhat on the fence about breastfeeding. Preventing necrotizing enterocolitis in babies is an important benefit of breastfeeding, but it is hard to be inspired by this fact when you *don't know what necrotizing enterocolitis is* (it is a very serious and horrible infection of the intestinal tract). Making a child smarter and happier, by contrast, is something that for most of us is much easier to grasp and much more motivating. If the message about the intellectual and behavioral benefits for breastfeeding starts to get watered down, one might worry, we lose the "hook" that is most likely to motivate moms to want to breastfeed as long as they can, thereby losing the many other less sexy medical benefits of breastfeeding in the process.

Yet there remains much upon which to base an enthusiastic, if not righteous, promotion for breastfeeding. Despite all of the intense scrutiny and controlling for many other complicating factors, associations continue to be found between improved child verbal abilities and longer durations of breastfeeding. Further, there is some evidence that these gains may be particularly pronounced in families from more disadvantaged backgrounds who are also incidentally the folks who are less likely to try breastfeeding on their own without additional help and motivation. All in all, this doesn't sound much like a balloon whose air is being removed, but rather a message that could be supportively publicized as one of many things young parents can do to help build healthy brains.

## It Depends—Breastfeeding and Intelligence

### General Summary

There is evidence that longer a duration of breastfeeding is linked to modest increases in child intellectual ability, particularly in verbal skills. Previous claims of large IQ gains, in addition to benefits related to child behavior and security, however, are likely due to other factors that often are associated with mothers who breastfeed.

| "It Depends" Factor | Adjustment |
| --- | --- |
| Maternal diet | Intellectual gains associated with breastfeeding may be more pronounced among women who consume healthy omega-3 fatty acids found in foods such cold water fish. |
| Family socioeconomic status and IQ | Intellectual gains associated with breastfeeding may be more pronounced among families from more disadvantaged backgrounds and among children with relatively lower IQs. |

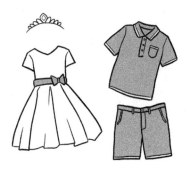

# 7

# Blue, Pink, or Yellow?

## How Parents Can Affect Gender Development

Girl or boy? This often is the very first question a new or expecting parent gets asked. In the old days, new babies were announced with cigars wrapped in pink or blue ribbons. These days, however, it is not only the cigars that have come under scrutiny, but the ribbons as well. As more and more individuals describe their inner feelings of being male or female in expanded terms that don't match up with the simple boy versus girl assignment at birth, many parents are beginning to question their role in shaping a child's gender development. Are we, as parents, essentially spectators to a parade governed by genetics and hormones, or are we sculptors with powers to influence not only our children's gender-based behaviors and attitudes but their very identity as male, female, or somewhere in between? This chapter will explore the science around gender expression and identity formation and the various sources that determine it. The focus will be not only on how parents *respond* to some of the early manifestations of their child's gender identity and expression but also the ways we may actually *create* that identity with subtle, or not so subtle, cues.

Four-year-old Jordan is often called a "tomboy." She loves sports and has asked to keep her hair short. Recently, she's even started to express a dislike of clothes with too many flowers or butterflies on them. Her parents have tried their best to avoid confining her to typical gender stereotypes but haven't

Chapter illustrations drawn by Jaq Fagnant

*Parenting Made Complicated.* David C. Rettew, Oxford University Press (2021). © Oxford University Press.
DOI: 10.1093/oso/9780197550977.003.0007

really thought twice about using pronouns other than "she" and "her" when talking with or referring to Jordan. At a recent family gathering, an 18-year-old cousin of Jordan wonders whether Jordan might be *nonbinary* and suggests that they explore more gender options for Jordan as kindergarten approaches. The cousin asks about their pronoun use and the school bathroom that the parents encourage her to use and implies that Jordan may come to feel rejected and invalidated by the parents if they are not more proactive in their acceptance of Jordan's emerging gender nonconformity.

Some readers might be a little surprised to see this chapter in the infancy section of the book. Infants, after all, are oblivious to gender issues until later, right? Experts do often claim that babies are blissfully unaware of gender until about the age of 3, when there is a rapid uptick in the amount of preschool-age brain power paid to the subject. Sure, a little girl might have been dressed in flowery clothes for years, but it is not until later that she starts really to be aware, take notice, and make judgments about people being male or female, even if those judgments can get thrown off track by a woman wearing pants or a man with long hair. The preschool years are also the time when sex differences with regard to behavior begin to emerge—smaller with regard to things like temperamental traits such as activity level (boys are somewhat higher) and much larger for things like toy preferences, which can be evident as early as an infant's first birthday.[1,2] Classrooms also can start to look more segregated by gender with boys and girls often hanging out in different parts of the room and doing different activities. One estimate found that by the end of kindergarten, children are only spending 9% of their playtime with opposite sex peers.[3,4] By around age 6 or 7, children have supposedly achieved "gender constancy," meaning that they come to understand that their gender (or really their sex in more precise terms) is fixed and does not change. But this older concept is now being questioned by those who believe the gender journey can continue well past this time, especially in societies that don't suppress it. Indeed, as children develop ever more advanced cognitive skills, they are able to hold more nuanced and less dogmatic views about what gender does and does not mean for themselves and others.

But before getting too far ahead of ourselves, the reason the gender development chapter is being discussed along with things like daycare and sleep training is that even if infants are relatively oblivious to the idea of gender, *you*, the parents, are not. Rather, gender considerations in parenting come up quite early, with decisions needing to be made even before a child is born. After the ultrasound revealing the sex of the fetus, many parents are ready to jump all-in to create that magical pink princess-themed nursery for their new daughter or that bright blue baseball–dump truck–dinosaur motif for their expected son. But is that really just a fun and innocent celebration of new life or a box that will constrain a child's view of themselves and others for years to come?

Lisa and Tony are expecting their first child. During a prenatal visit, the couple find out that they are "having a boy." Both of them are excited, and Tony is eager to start designing the nursery with bold colors and a baseball theme to reflect Tony's lifelong love of the game that he is eager to share with his new son. Lisa, however, expresses some hesitation about pushing male stereotypes right from birth and wonders about a more neutral-looking room. Tony is very skeptical that the decorations in a bedroom have any impact whatsoever on the development of this future shortstop for the Oakland A's, but he is willing to bring up this question to their obstetrician at the next visit.

## Some Terminology

Gender development is a broad concept that encompasses the processes through which children come not only to define themselves and those around them in terms of gender but also the pathway toward understanding what being male or female actually means. Gender development also includes ways children acquire particular behaviors and ideas that society views as being at least somewhat specific to girls or boys. But before plunging into how all this happens, it might be useful first to define some important terms. The language when it comes to gender development and related constructs can get confusing and continues to evolve, so some clear definitions might help. One good source is the website for GLAAD (formerly the Gay and Lesbian Alliance Against Defamation).[5] Box 7.1 describes some important terms that will be used throughout this chapter.

Chief among these is the difference between sex and gender. A child's sex, which develops from one's genetic composition (usually having two X chromosomes for females and an X and a Y chromosome for males) is assigned at birth based on one's external genital anatomy. Gender expression refers to the degree to which someone's outward behavior and choices fall in line with conventions of masculinity and femininity while gender identity, by contrast, deals more with the internal sense of *being* male, female or somewhere along a continuum. Concepts surrounding gender have a lot more to do with one's brain than external anatomy.

## Box 7.1  Selected Terms in Gender Development

- Sex: the classification of someone (usually male or female) at birth based on one's external anatomy
- Gender identity: an individual's internal sense of being male, female or somewhere in the middle
- Gender expression: the manifestations of one's gender through things like clothing, language, mannerisms, and preferences
- Sexual orientation: this describes the gender of a person's romantic or sexual attraction
- Trans or transgender: Someone who's gender identity and/or expression does not match their assigned sex
- Gender dysphoria: a feeling of discomfort, anxiety, or even anger about one's assigned sex at birth
- Cisgender: An individual whose gender identity matches their assigned sex
- Gender non-conforming, Non Binary, Genderqueer: A more general term to describe people whose gender expression and identity do not fit traditional distinctions.
- Gender fluid: A dynamic state in which a person's gender identity fluctuates over time

Liam is now 5 years old. While he was born with typical male anatomy, there have been indications that he is quite uncomfortable with his designation as a boy since he could walk and talk. His play preferences from the start have gravitated to more typically "girl" toys, and he has resisted cutting his hair. At age 3, he asked to be able to wear a dress and at age 4 told his parents that he is a "girl on the inside." More recently, he asked to be called Evie instead of Liam. These preferences have been challenging for the parents, especially for Liam's father who has occasionally become angry with Liam and anyone else who he feels has been "encouraging this stuff." As a result, Liam has recently become more irritable and sad. At school, he is starting to get teased by some of his classmates for his feelings, which is making Liam feel even worse about himself. The parents are getting very concerned and take Liam to their pediatrician for advice.

Some terms that get used in discussions of gender status and definitions change over time. Realizing this, I apologize now for using terminology that by the time this book goes to print could already be outdated. Discussions about gender expression and identity can also evoke a lot of strong emotions from many different political directions. People with gender-nonconforming beliefs and behaviors have been the target of intense bullying, ridicule, and violence, as will be discussed in more detail soon. While perspectives have changed over the years, there still remains a long way to go. Going forward, the hope here is to be able to take an honest look at the science on gender development while keeping in mind the various ways that this science can be used and misused for ideological purposes.

## Gender Identity, Genes, and Hormones

The degree to which someone acts in a more masculine or feminine way is not considered to be a classic temperament or personality trait. Terms like macho or girly are common and convey ideas that most people understand, but most researchers have preferred to leave out gender identity in their temperament or personality frameworks and focus instead on more specific and observable traits such as assertiveness or emotionality without the baggage of having to layer gender on top of them. Nevertheless, a person's defined gender does possess some trait-like features and can be a core aspect of a child's sense of self. As a result, it is worth spending a little time on how gender identity is formed and what forces determine it.

While much emphasis is placed on the way that parents, peers, and culture can affect a young child's gender development, it's important to remember that a lot of other influences are at work at the same time. Male XY fetuses compared to female XX fetuses are exposed to different concentrations of hormones such as testosterone and estrogen during critical developmental periods in utero, right after birth, and, of course, around puberty. These hormones not only impact organs such as ovaries, breasts, and testes but the brain as well. Interestingly the timing of these effects on different organs can vary. While the presence or absence of hormones like testosterone very early in fetal development have profound impacts on the development of male or female genitalia, the sex specific influences on the brain occur later in pregnancy.[6] This difference suggests the possibility of some degree of independence between the biology driving one's sex and the biology driving one's gender.[7]

Twin studies that compare how similar identical twins are to fraternal twins consistently show a sizable but not certainly not overwhelming influence of genetics on gender expression and stereotypical masculine or feminine behavior. In one study of nearly 4000 preschool-age twins, the proportion of genetic influence on scores for a rating scale that measured the amount of gender-typical behaviors was found to be 34% for boys and 57% for girls.[8]

There are also certain situations and medical conditions that can offer clues about the relative importance of early biological influences in shaping gender identity and expression. One involves infants and young children who are born male but then suffer an injury or medical mishap to their penis that leads the parents in some cases to decide to raise the child as female. Probably the most famous case, and one of the most tragic, was of David Reimer who was raised as a girl after a circumcision accident.[9] Despite his parents' efforts, which they based on the medical opinions they received at the time, Reimer's female identity never fit with regard to his play, dress, or sexual attractions. After learning the truth of his early history, David decided to change his identity to male but continued to struggle emotionally even after marrying a woman and adopting children. He eventually died by suicide at age 38. While this story is a compelling one that speaks to the power of genetics and early biology, it turns out not to be very typical. A review of over 70 individuals with similar circumstances found that many of these children grew up to be fairly comfortable in their female identity, although many did manifest more male-associated behaviors and preferences.[10]

Another condition worth mentioning is congenital adrenal hyperplasia—a genetic disorder that can result in female fetuses being exposed to higher than average levels of male hormones or androgens. These children are mostly raised as girls and undergo surgery to feminize their external genitalia, which can sometimes be more ambiguous. Studies of genetically female individuals with congenital adrenal hyperplasia again show higher amounts of "boyish" behavior, but the vast majority of these children identify as female.[11] Increasingly, however, surgical procedures for infants and children with atypical genitalia or intersex conditions have become more controversial. Many individuals, some of whom have had these procedures, have criticized these surgeries and the gender assignments that come with them, in the process raising important questions about who should make gender decisions such as these and when.[12]

More common are cases of opposite sex fraternal (dizygotic) twins. Here again, the female twin will be exposed to somewhat higher levels of androgens due to the presence of a male twin in the same uterus. A complicating wrinkle in these families is that these female twins are often brought up with the full repertoire of toys in the household from dolls to dump trucks, thereby lessening the impact of more stereotypical gender behavior being due to a lack of choices. Studies of opposite-sex twins tend not to find clear evidence of more masculine behavior in these female twins, although some subtle differences have been documented.[4,13]

There are also lines of evidence showing that some aspects of gender differentiation is beginning much earlier than the conventional wisdom of age 2 to

3. Newborns in only their first week of life can show behavioral differences between boys and girls, with girls showing more interest in human faces and boys showing more interest in mechanical objects.[14] Sex-based differences in behavior are also found among other species of animals that don't paint their offspring's bedrooms in particular colors. Male monkeys, for example, prefer to play with more physically active things like balls and toy cars while female monkeys are more like to play with dolls.[15] I'm still waiting on the study of male and female monkeys when it comes to watching football games.

In terms of the brain, differences between men and women are subtle—and, to some, remarkably so for something as fundamental as one's sex. This topic, it turns out, is an area of some debate within the neuroscience community, with some researchers reporting essentially no reliable overall differences between male and female brains[16] while other studies do show that some specific regions, like the hippocampus or amygdala, being, on average, relatively larger or smaller in males versus females. Interestingly, some of these sex differences are evident only at specific ages.[7] Yes, the brains of males tend to be a little larger than those of females, but variations in human brain size don't correlate very well with attributes such as intelligence or a strong wit. All said, while the social media arguments and cheap cocktail party jabs about gender and brain anatomy will invariably continue, it is probably safe to say that in the brain there is nothing that is the equivalent of a Y chromosome—that is, some structure that clearly differentiates males from females. Further, studies of people with gender dysphoria continue to be inconsistent on finding evidence that their brains look more closely like those of their affirmed gender than those of their assigned sex.[17]

In total, these data speak to the reality that a solid portion of gender stereotypical behavior and gender identity is "hard-wired" into the brain. Politically, however, this insight can cut both ways as it supports the authenticity of not only the child exhibiting very traditional gender-based behavior and identity but also the child voicing feelings of gender incongruence or dysphoria. After my first two boys were born, their mother and I were determined not to be those parents pushing macho gender stereotypes on their male children. To prove it, we bought them not just a dollhouse but a *really nice* dollhouse with genuine wooden furniture and realistic looking rooms. We got it with the idea that this would be an equally attractive alternative for their play to complement the more boy-typical toys that were there as well. And while I can't eliminate the possibility that they were receiving more subtle signals about the "proper" ways boys should play, I never saw that dollhouse being used for anything other than an escape shelter for action toys fleeing dinosaur attacks or a great landing pad for airborne monster trucks.

## Beyond Genes and Hormones

Genes and hormones are certainly not the end of the story when it comes to gender development. Parents, teachers, peers, the media, and many other environmental sources can conspire to turn small genetically influenced differences into big ones, if not create differences that weren't there in the first place.[4] As was recently argued in an entire special edition of the *Journal of Adolescent Health*, a child's gender obviously has huge implications for their future in ways that go well beyond the color and style of their clothing. Educational attainment, risk of sexual violence, and even life expectancy are all related to gender at varying degrees across the globe.[18,19] Societies, of course, differ on the size of their "gender gap" when it comes to things like political empowerment and economic opportunities. According to the World Economic Forum, which publishes the Global Gender Gap report each year, 2017 was the first year since they started studying this that the global gender gap actually increased worldwide.[20] From their calculation for 144 countries, Iceland followed by Norway emerged as the countries with the smallest gender gap while the largest gap was found for Yemen and Pakistan. The United States came in 49th.

For this chapter, however, the main question is not so much whether or not an authoritarian society can force gender stereotypes and oppress individuals from authentically expressing themselves (I think we all know the answer to that one), but the degree to which a loosening of the grip on gender assumptions and expectations by parents and others leads to a less binary distribution of traits, attitudes, preferences, and perhaps even of gender identity across a population. Sure, there may be widening cultural consensus around the idea that little girls should not be indoctrinated into the belief that they are delicate and subordinate while boys should not be bombarded with expectations that they should be invulnerable and dominant, but how far should a well-meaning parent take this? Is that pink on the wall of a newborn girl's bedroom really setting in motion a train of societal instructions about what it means to be a girl, or is it just paint? To get some answers, we now look at some of the research that examines the capacity of a child's environment to shape gender development.

Even without parents really trying, one important factor when it comes to gender development of young children is actually siblings, especially older ones. One study that was designed to look at the effect of having a male co-twin on girls between the ages of 3 and 8 found little when it came to the co-twin but more of an impact for girls who had an older brother. These girls showed more interest in traditionally male toys and were also more involved in athletics.[21] Peers are also an important influence even at young ages. One older but still fascinating study of preschoolers who entered a room of various "boy" and "girl" toys found that the amount of time a child spent playing with "opposite sex" toys significantly dropped if another child was in the room.[22]

When it comes to parental behavior, a number of slightly deceptive studies involving some degree of trickery demonstrate clearly that adults behave differently toward male versus female infants and young children (or what they think are male and female children) and make different interpretations of a child's behavior based on their perceived gender.[23,24] Male infants and toddlers, for example, tend to receive more physically oriented play from adults while their female counterparts get more verbal interactions.[4] Consequently, when we hear things like little boys are *just* better at sports or little girls *just* are more verbal, it is easy to chalk everything up to genetic destiny and forget that there very well could be an important role in how the environment cultivated those particular traits and abilities. One great example of this is the often-mentioned phenomenon that babies tend to respond preferentially to adult female faces or voices—data that are sometimes invoked to justify why it is the mom who naturally should be home with the kids. One study that tested this hypothesis indeed found it to be true, but only for infants in which the mother was already the primary caregiver. For the infants in which the father spent the most time with the baby, the trend was reversed.[25]

There also is plenty of evidence showing that parents react differently when their young child reaches for a gender typical versus atypical toy.[26] This difference is especially present when it comes to dads reacting to their sons playing with "girl" toys. The kids, of course, become aware of these reactions in their parents,[27] and from there it is not too difficult to guess what many eager-to-please preschoolers do to secure some good play time with Mom and Dad. Over time, kids tend to get better at the activities they do a lot, which leads further to the snowball effect of small, more innate-based differences becoming stronger. These differences in play can also translate into the types of more general skills, such as verbal, spatial, or motor abilities, that get honed with practice.

All these research findings have led people to wonder what then happens when a child's environment backs off on its expectations and nudging as to how little boys and girls are supposed to think and behave. In Sweden, a number of "gender-neutral" preschools have sprung up in which teachers actively try to counteract gender assumptions and stereotypes and even avoid using gendered language. Dolls and trucks are interspersed on the shelves and teachers work hard to avoid treating girls and boys differently when it comes to their tone of voice or the way rules are enforced. In a study that compared children in some of these preschools to those in more traditional ones, the researchers found that children in the gender-neutral preschools where less stereotypical when it came to ascribing certain toys or clothing as being for boys or girls and were more interested in playing with an unfamiliar child of the other gender.[28]

The size of these effects, however, were rather small. Furthermore, for some other variables measured, like the tendency to want to play with a same gender playmate, no significant difference between the two types of schools was found at all.

The relatively minor effects seen in studies like this could be interpreted as more evidence for the hard-wired theory of gender development. On the other hand, one could also argue that the intervention itself was also on a small scale. The classroom environment may have changed, but kids even in gender-neutral schools get exposed to more traditional gender-based pressures from many other sources. To get a better idea of what things might look like when gender neutrality is taken to the next level, we need to go beyond the classroom to efforts that encompass the totality of the child's environment. One place to look is the relatively recent phenomenon of gender-neutral parenting (GNP) or, to use the popular media term, *theybies*. In this approach, which can vary from family to family with regard to intensity, parents do their best to avoid *anything* that would push gender stereotypes onto their children and, in some cases, don't even reveal the sex of their child to anyone (not even the child) for as long as possible. Gender pronouns are avoided, and these children are free to choose their clothing or toys regardless of its gender label. Why go to this extreme? Proponents of GNP often believe that this practice not only helps kids who will go on to be gender-nonconforming feel more secure and accepted but, for those kids who end up developing a cisgender identity, helps them to become more open minded and accepting of others. Related to some of the recently described research on how people behave differently around children based on their perceived gender, the method also keeps other adults from projecting their own gender biases onto these kids. Some parents see the approach less about being gender *neutral* per se and more about giving children the space and time to find their own true place on the gender spectrum.

Many people, myself included, are very interested to find out how children raised in a GNP approach turn out. Are these kids more likely to display less gender stereotypical traits and behaviors? Will they be less sexist and more embracing of LGBTQ individuals? Will they be more likely to develop a transgender or at least a nonbinary gender identity later in life? There are lots of good question here but, unfortunately, little systematic research on this topic. Anecdotal reports and articles do indeed suggest that these children, at least as they go through the elementary school years, do show a broader range of gender expression regarding things like clothing, toys, and play preferences.[29] More rigorous studies, however, are lacking and time will tell when it comes to how persistent these behaviors are and the degree to which they transcend into the deeper level of gender identity and the core sense of being male or female, the topic we focus on next.

## Gender Identity

Recall that gender expression reflects an individual's gender-related behavior when it comes to things like mannerisms and preferences while gender identity refers to someone's inner feelings about where they belong on the male/female spectrum. One important topic that remains inadequately understood is the very imperfect correspondence between these two related constructs of gender expression and gender identity. While it is true that individuals who show more gender incongruent expression are more likely to have a nonbinary gender identity, the correlation is far from perfect. Plenty of kids who are assigned female at birth, for example, embrace more "tomboy" characteristics and may even come out as gay with regards to sexual orientation without ever feeling as though their gender identity is anything other than female. Similarly, other children raised as girls can come to see themselves as transgender while still choosing to exhibit a lot of more stereotypical feminine behavior and appearances. Exactly what a person is sensing in themselves that propels them to affirm that their gender-nonconforming expression is part of a larger gender-nonconforming identity (i.e., that they actually *are not* the gender they were assigned at birth) can be hard to describe, even among people experiencing it. Finding something in the brain that corresponds to these related concepts has been murkier still.

This relative independence between gender expression and gender identity means that we can't assume that the forces that affect gender expression, both genetic and environmental, have similar impacts on gender identity and the degree to which a person intrinsically feels male or female. It is often the case, for example, that engaging little girls in sports and more active play changes preferences, ability, and confidence levels about these activities later in life while having no effect at all on their identity as being female. Indeed, media campaigns such as "Play Like a Girl"[30] are built around the premise that society has no business carving out things like being a badass athlete as part of the male identity. Yet even the relatively progressive thinking Pope Francis has voiced concern about the ability of adults to *push* children toward a transgender identity through the "ideological colonization" contained in viewing gender identity as something intrinsically less binary and more discoverable for each person.[31] More recently, a significant controversy has been raised regarding adolescents who have unofficially been labeled as having "rapid onset gender dysphoria." According to some parents of these youth, these are older children and adolescents, most of whom with little to no early history of seeing themselves as transgender or nonbinary, who quickly become so supposedly based on the influence of social media and peers. A not particularly rigorous research paper in 2018, based on a SurveyMonkey tally given to the *parents only*, describes for the first time a group of adolescents and young adults who experience a gender dysphoria "outbreak" after friends or online acquaintances expressed gender dysphoric or transgender views.[32e2] A large percentage of this sample also had been diagnosed with a psychiatric disorder. The controversy, not unexpectedly, comes from the insinuation that at least some transgender individuals develop their gender identity as more of a fad through social contagion or as a maladaptive coping mechanism to emotional-behavioral problems. The negative response to this paper was severe and its scientific shortcomings attacked to the point that the journal that published it, *PLoS One*, is now reviewing its publication process. The author's academic institution, Brown University, stopped featuring the study.[33] This backing away from the data, in turn, has created its own backlash by people concerned about the censorship of science that may be politically sensitive or inconvenient.

These heated debates clearly reflect different conclusions people have already reached on how gender identity is determined. If you believe that gender identity is driven by genetics and neurobiology that is mostly beyond anyone's control, then any drift that occurs in a single individual or a group of individuals in response to a society's loosening of rigid gender expectations reflects a migration to a "truer" set point—free of the bondage of cultural stereotypes. If, however, you believe that popular trends, social media, peer pressure, and of course, parental encouragement can at least temporarily "confuse" a young person into endorsing a false and, for most people, superficial gender identity, then it is easy to view these new perspectives on gender as creating a lot of needless trouble and unrest.

Thus, we now shift to look at what science knows about transgender and nonbinary individuals with an eye especially toward the degree to which parental actions can affect both their child's actual gender identity and their child's well-being. According to a 2018 study, about 3% of adolescents describe themselves as transgender or gender-nonconforming.[34] In younger samples, rates of gender "atypical" behavior or expressions of gender dissatisfaction are even more common. In a previously mentioned Dutch study of 7- and 10-year olds, approximately 3% of boys and 5% of girls often behave like the "opposite" sex while parents rate that about 1% of kids actually voice the preference to be the gender not assigned to them at birth.[35] The vast majority of these kids do not go on to identify as transgender, although it is unclear if that is because they genuinely no longer continue to have those feelings or because external forces drive those thoughts underground. A sizable percentage of youth who express clear and persistent gender dysphoria, maybe up to 80% for boys but probably less for girls, do go on to have a homosexual or bisexual orientation while usually keeping a cisgender identity.[36]

Unfortunately, many gender-nonconforming youth struggle with their mental health. Depression, suicide, substance abuse, and other mental health problems are significantly higher among LGBTQ children and adolescents compared to their non-LGBTQ peers.[37–39] While the acknowledgment of these associations is not controversial, what remains debatable is the cause. In the eyes of many, the emotional-behavioral turmoil facing many of these individuals is *completely* explained by the well-documented bullying, abuse, and rejection that so many gay and gender-nonconforming people are forced to endure.[40] While few deny this sad reality, others maintain that, in addition, there is mental suffering that comes more intrinsically from the realization of a mismatch between ones assigned sex and one's affirmed gender. This debate is reflected in the shifting definitions over the years of gender nonconformity as a psychiatric diagnosis. Previously, the term *gender identity disorder* applied to someone who displayed persistent gender "atypical" expression or a belief that their actual gender was different than their birth assigned sex.[41] In 2013, the powers that be officially changed the term to *gender dysphoria* to reflect that the diagnosis would no longer apply to someone who was comfortable with their nonbinary identity and should only be used for people who experience distress and impairment from this discontinuity.

In an effort to test these two hypotheses on the cause of mental health problems in gender-nonconforming youth, an influential study from 2016 examined a group of younger transgender children between the ages of 3 and 12 whose families fully supported their affirmed gender.[42] These were children who "persistently, insistently, and consistently" identified as the gender opposite of their assigned sex at birth and had already transitioned to their affirmed gender both at home and at school. In looking at the mental health of this relatively unique sample, the researchers found no increased levels of depression and only slight elevations in anxiety relative to a control group. The authors concluded that mental health problems are not directly the result of a transgender identity and can be avoided when a person feels validated and supported by parents and others. In response to data such as these, there has been a shift in the approach that many primary care and mental health clinicians take when working with gender-nonconforming youth: less gentle prodding of a child to get them "back" to a cisgender identity and more emphasis on encouraging adults to support a child's stated gender and to protect them from the stigma, shame, and outright abuse that can be directed the child's way.

Yet herein lies the dilemma for many parents. In being aware of some of these mental health statistics surrounding gender-nonconforming youth and the harsh realities that too many of these kids face, even a loving nonfascist parent might think it best to *accept* their child's gender nonconformity if it comes up but not necessarily *encourage* gender nonconformity from the start under the premise that promoting it might actually *create* a gender identity that subjects their child to a lot of otherwise preventable hostility from an intolerant world. A parent, in trying to balance these two objectives, may certainly not want to reject and criticize a child's interest in gender-nonconforming clothes or activities, but that's not the same thing as actively fostering more gender fluidity from the start as is done with GNP.

All this, of course, hinges on how much sway parents have on child gender identity in the first place. To find out, different lines of evidence could be quite useful. As we saw earlier, studies of twins are a good place to look. One study of twin children between the ages of 3 and 17 found that the heritability for scores on a gender identity rating scale was an impressive 62% with the remaining environmental component being of the "unshared" type—which means environmental factors that tend to make children in the same family more different from each other rather than more similar.[43] This result would seem to suggest that the ability of parents to create a household environment that has a major impact on gender identity is limited. Similarly, another study of over 20,000 twins that measured "cross" gender behavior in children aged 7 and 10 found even larger heritabilties of up to 70%.[35] In reviewing the published studies on twins who were concordant or discordant for that older diagnosis of gender identity disorder, the authors found an overall rate of concordance of 39% for identical (monozygotic) twins versus 0% for fraternal (dizygotic) twins, again suggesting a significant effect of genetics.[44] Some specific genes have also been linked to gender dysphoria, although like in most everything related to behavior, no single gene explains that much.[45]

It is also useful to hear the stories of individuals who desire gender-affirming medical interventions in the form of hormonal treatment and surgery. In this group, significant feelings of gender incongruence have typically been present for many years and continue to be stable into adolescence and adulthood.[46] In a study of 55 transgender adults who underwent gender-affirming treatment, none reported regret over their decision.[47] These accounts paint a very different picture than the portrayal of gender identity as something whimsical and capricious that can change with a persuasive social media post. This is not to say that peers or the media can't influence aspects of gender development or that there cannot exist individuals whose full realization of their gender does not reach total awareness until later in life but that overall gender identity is a tree with deep roots unlikely to be pushed around for too long by the breezes of pop culture and fads.

Finally, we stand to learn quite a bit from children who have been raised under a GNP approach. While I am not aware of any major research study of these kids, publications will invariably begin to surface over the next several years. My expectation is that most of the "theybies" will turn out pretty much like their more genderized peers with most being quite healthy physically and mentally and some struggling. It would not surprise me if many children raised under more GNP conditions develop a more nuanced, dimensional view of gender that helps them accept, even celebrate, the wide diversity of gender expression and identity that is revealing itself today. However, I'd be surprised if the majority of them developed a transgender identity in the long run. Indeed, as is often the case with children, I'm sure a few will also completely rebel against the best wishes of their parents and encase themselves with pink princess castles and blue dinosaur jet fighter designs just to annoy them.

## Summary

Overall, then, there is fairly convincing evidence that gender development is shaped by a number of different factors. Some of these, like genetics and exposure to various hormones before birth, are difficult for parents to control yet can have real effects with regard to things like temperamental traits such as how physically active a child is or other characteristics like play style or toy preferences. Yet the science also shows rather strongly that gender development can also be influenced by the environment and the many ways that gender-based attitudes and conventions work their way into the everyday fabric of child-rearing. These influences may not usually be strong enough to change a child's fundamental view of themselves as male or female, but it can have quite an impact on the way a child sees their particular traits and interests as valuable and accepted.

After a discussion with their obstetrician, Lisa and Tony find some middle ground when it comes to their nursery planning, and they both agree they don't want to box in their new son's identity before he is even born. Baseball decorations will be part of the nursery decorations but typically male themes will not dominate the room. The color scheme will also be more neutral than the standard boy blue. After all, Lisa points out, the A's team colors do happen to be green and gold.

For parents, all this boils down to the reality that we have significant but certainly not unlimited power to introduce, prohibit, reinforce, or discourage actions and thoughts in our children that conform to gender stereotypes or break the mold. Not all of our gender-related aspirations as parents will get adopted in our children's development, and, for some, the momentum of genetics and biology will reign supreme no matter what we do, but for most children it is certainly fair to say that parents are far more than objective bystanders when it comes to our child's journey in gender development. In trying to translate all these studies into practical information, one might distill this research into the overall recommendation that, as parents, you would do well to avoid imposing rigid gender-based stereotypes on your children from the start. From there, you can *follow your child's lead* when it comes to their own gender identity and expression. Accomplishing this approach will require an open and curious mind, but as of yet there is not evidence that a completely gender neutral approach is essential to help children understand that their assigned sex at birth should mean little when it comes to their inclinations, their appearance, and, most important, their potential.

Jordan's parents think carefully about what the cousin said about being more assertive in supporting Jordan's presumed nonbinary gender identity. They ultimately decide, however, not to change course. They will continue to support Jordan's sense of gender wherever it takes them without getting out ahead of it and assuming something that may or may not be there. They have age-appropriate discussions of human bodies and the difference between sex and gender. The parents continue to refer to Jordan as "she," pending further instructions. Five years later, Jordan asks to join the football team, arguing that its unavailability to girls is in violation of her rights. A major controversy ensues in the community.

## It Depends

### Gender Typical Behavior

When it comes to "it depends" factors for how best parents can support their child's gender development, there isn't much in the published literature about reacting differently to kids with different temperaments. Nevertheless, there remain other factors deserving comment, even if the overall conclusions tend to double down on the main recommendations rather than sending you in a different direction.

Back in chapter 3, you heard the somewhat odd-sounding advice that parents may want to take stock of what types of parenting behavior comes most naturally and then consider the possibility of taking a few steps in the *opposite* direction. In somewhat the same vein, it is worth a few moments for you to take a look at your own behaviors and attitudes when it comes to gender and think how this may be coming across to your kids. Since a parent is often the most powerful and salient role model of a child, you are typically your kid's de facto *standard* for what gender means. As such, there can be real benefits to getting the topic a bit more out in the open. This could be especially true if a child's early gender tendencies don't line up with what they are seeing in their parent. A more effeminate son of a very typically masculine father, for example, might be feeling a bit uneasy about his emerging sense of himself and might need more deliberate affirmations and shows of support. Likewise, more traditional cisgender mothers might need to take an extra step or two to convince a daughter that the acceptable gender landscape for girls is broader than it may appear.

The same holds true for "it depends" factors regarding how gender typical a *child* is leaning. While, of course, one of the main themes here is to embrace a child's gender development wherever it is, children who naturally seem prone to very gender typical behaviors and attitudes need to be given the *opportunity* to show aspects of themselves that are not so stereotypical in an effort to prevent them from getting overly swept up in the tide of their own gender-based momentum. Some of the research previously reviewed in this chapter illustrates quite well how the world responds differently to children based on their gender. For kids who display more typical gender roles from the start, it may be doubly easy to fall into this pattern and forget that your son who only seems to want to engage in battle games might, with the proper encouragement, also enjoy playing family once in a while. Similarly, while there may be nothing at all wrong with a little girl who legitimately wants to dress up as a princess all the time, there's no rule that says that she can't be the princess who also hits the cover off the baseball at Little League.

## Intensity of Gender Incongruence

When it comes to the question of how a parent best reacts to their child gender development, one crucial "it depends" factor that is starting to show up in research studies is the child's intensity and persistence of their gender identity feelings and beliefs. In particular, children who express strong and more enduring views about being transgender or nonbinary can be prone to emotional struggles when these feelings are invalidated or outright resisted by parents and other important parts of a child's environment. The previously mentioned study that demonstrated how well adjusted transgender children can be when they are in a supportive household sends an important message. No, parents don't need to be rushing to the principle to advocate that their 5-year-old son who likes to play with dolls use the girls bathroom, but young children who voice more persistent and pervasive gender incongruence are going to need your support and may be vulnerable to mental health problems if they perceive you as disapproving and rejecting of who they are. Some of these kids will continue to have strong feelings of gender incongruence as they get older and some will not, but regardless, these children will greatly benefit from knowing that their parents are in their corner, even if too many others are not.

> Liam's parents are told that their child is voicing clear indications of a non-binary gender identity and is showing signs of psychological harm by not having their feelings accepted either at home or at school. The pediatrician tells the parents that it is impossible to say at this point whether or not this gender identity will persist but that for Liam's sake there needs to be a major move toward helping them feel better about how who they is. While the parents worry about continued hardships down the road for Liam, they agree to change course at home and ask to meet with the school about ways to better support Liam there. The parents begin to use the name Evie and the pronoun "they" and push the school to do the same. They decide to allow Evie to wear a dress to school. When the father drops Evie off at school that first day, he wears one too in solidarity.

## It Depends—Gender Development

**General Summary**

While genetics and hormonal exposure play large roles in the development of both gender expression and gender identity, parents also possess influence particularly related to a child's attitudes about gender and to a child's opportunity to pursue their full range of interests and preferences.

| "It Depends" Factor | Adjustment |
|---|---|
| More gender stereotypical children | These children may be particularly likely to have their gender stereotypical behavior reinforced by others. Parents may need to take more deliberate steps to ensure that they have opportunities to express less gender stereotypical ideas and traits. |
| Gender-nonconforming children | These children are especially vulnerable to abuse and bullying as well as feeling unaccepted by others. Parents need to be especially mindful that any "nudging" toward more cisgender expression and identity may come across as rejecting. |

# PART 3

# TODDLERS AND PRESCHOOLERS

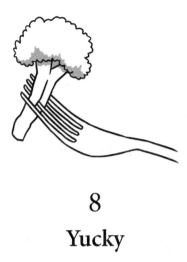

# 8

# Yucky

## Finding Solutions for Picky Eaters

As they say in the classic movie *A Christmas Story*—every family has a kid who won't eat. For most parents, a child's picky and selective eating is a source of considerable irritation that transforms what otherwise would be an enjoyable and relaxing meal into an epic battle of wits—complete with nags, rewards, negotiations, praise, and empty threats that a child will remain 3-feet tall for the rest of her life. And, indeed, in some cases, there can be very real problems related to nutritional status and growth. Most kids, however, miraculously seem to be able to subsist just fine on a revolving rotation that consists entirely of chicken nuggets, pizza, grilled cheese, and French fries, although this reality alone isn't enough for most parents to justify giving up the fight.

In the movie, little Randy is made to sit at the table until he finishes his meal—a common practice at the time that remains etched in the memories of many parents today. But today's time-crunched world doesn't seem to allow for the luxury of sitting around a table for 2 hours waiting for a preschooler to eat their mashed potatoes, so instead the more common practice among parents who remain committed to their child's nutritional health is a constant barrage of reminders and encouragement to eat while a scrumptious dessert is dangled for good kids who clean their plate. Sandwiches get painstakingly sculpted and crafted into cats or stars, and vegetables are secretly snuck into smoothies like something out of a Russian spy novel. When that doesn't work, parents become debate masters, trying to apply perfectly good and perfectly useless logic to the table ala, "You love ketchup and ketchup is made from tomatoes so why can't you

Chapter illustrations drawn by Jaq Fagnant

*Parenting Made Complicated.* David C. Rettew, Oxford University Press (2021). © Oxford University Press.
DOI: 10.1093/oso/9780197550977.003.0008

just eat the tomato?!" or guilt mongers, telling their kids that children in whatever country is currently experiencing a massive food shortage would kill to have what is sitting right there on their child's plate.

It's exhausting work, this dog-and-pony show that so many parents end up having to perform to get a young child to consume even a small portion of green peas or unprocessed chicken. Even more exasperating is the fact that picky eating is one of those things that can creep up on parents after being lulled into a false sense of accomplishment. Typically, infants do pretty well as new foods are introduced. This apparent success is a delight to parents who marvel at their incredible skills of effortlessly being able to get their babies to eat green and brown mush with little to no resistance. At around age 2, however, things often head south in a hurry, as smug self-congratulations quickly morph into head-banging–level frustration (I'm talking about the parent here) over getting a toddler or preschooler to put down even a couple bites of something that she couldn't stop eating just a few weeks earlier.

> Ayden is a 4-year-old boy who had always been nervous and tentative around anything new. Food has been no exception. Since entering his toddler years, Ayden's parents have watched helplessly as his food choices have steadily shrunk to just a few generally carbohydrate-rich options. Now, most meals at home involve his parents making Ayden something different than the rest of the family. Ayden is growing normally, but it concerns and embarrasses the parents to see him be so fussy, especially in comparison to other children who seem to be able to consume whatever their parents serve without complaint.

## The Importance of Good Nutrition

Given these circumstances, it's no wonder that many mothers and fathers have found themselves bypassing the food battles altogether to become short-order cooks who provide a child's small repertoire of preferred foods on demand. Nuke up a few nuggets, plop a kid in front of an iPad, and a couple might even find some actual moments of peace and quiet to enjoy a meal to themselves. As for fruits and vegetables, there's always a tasty gummy vitamin to pick up some of the slack.

This strategy, however, is not without its hazards. The American Academy of Pediatrics has recently been urging both pediatricians and parents to step up their game when it comes to promoting good nutrition in early childhood given the increasing evidence that "failure to provide key nutrients during this critical period of brain development may result in lifelong deficits in brain function."[1p1] Even if a child is growing normally and shows no obvious sign of being malnourished, a very limited diet could mean that important nutrients are lacking. Looking from the more positive flip side, there is also evidence that providing good nutrition to disadvantaged youth can, in some cases, improve math, reading, and verbal skills to the point that the well-documented differences in these areas related to socioeconomic status are no longer detectable.[2] By "good nutrition," experts mean getting adequate and balanced amounts of both *macronutrients* (big categories of food like protein, fat, carbohydrates, etc.) and *micronutrients* (more specific things like Vitamin D and zinc we need in smaller amounts).

There, of course, is also a lot of concern lately about the *overconsumption* of many foods and the rising rates of obesity in children, with some of the sharpest increases being found among kids in the 2- to 5-year-old range.[3] According to recent estimates, approximately one in six youths in the United States is obese, which translates roughly into about 12.7 million children between the ages of 2 and 19.[4] The causes of obesity are many and involve both genetic and environmental factors, but there is little debate that our overreliance on processed and nutritionally suspect food is a major driver of these trends.[5] As eating habits in childhood lay the groundwork for dietary behavior later in life,[6] there are plenty of reasons for parents to try and help children learn to eat well from the start.

---

The parents of 5-year-old Ellie now dread mealtimes. The groans and complaints over being served anything that isn't highly processed have taken what once was pleasant and cherished family time to an experience that is now something to *get through*. Most of meal conversation now consists of trying to talk Ellie into eating a decent meal and how many more bites she needs to do before she can have dessert. Ellie has demonstrated some expert negotiation skills as she often prevails in getting her way over her battle-weary parents. Finally, after a particularly large meltdown over a single green bean, Ellie's mother wonders aloud that "there has got to be another way."

---

## Some Basic Facts

Given the varying levels of intensity children exhibit when it comes to restrictive eating habits, it's not surprising that the threshold of what should officially count as "picky" is difficult to establish. Indeed, it has been argued that, from an evolutionary perspective, a child's reluctance to try new foods may have had some survival advantages by protecting kids from gobbling down toxic berries or mushrooms.[7] These days, however, the presence of *food neophobia*, the term used by those in the know to describe children who are extremely wary of trying new foods, carries less of a selective advantage and seems to be switched off entirely for non-prehistoric foods that come in plastic wrappers.

Consensus over an official definition of picky or fussy eating continues to be absent, although most descriptions include an "inadequate" intake of both new and familiar foods due to rejection based on taste, texture, or, as many parents will acknowledge, the mere sight of it.[7,8] This then leads to a very limited diversity of acceptable foods, particularly when it comes to things like fruits and vegetables. Some researchers who study picky eating also find that many of these kids eat quite slowly and quickly get to the state of feeling "full."[9,10]

With this lack of clear benchmarks, it follows that the calculated rates of significant picky eating ranges widely for toddlers and preschoolers from anywhere between 5% and 60%.[7] In some studies, the rate peaks around age 3,[7,11] although this finding is not universal, and other studies show relatively stable levels across early childhood.[12] Contrary to popular lore, picky eating is a known phenomenon worldwide with some of highest rates being reported in countries such as Turkey and China.[12,13] The United States, however, does seem to report relatively high rates of fussy eating, up to around 50%,[14] in comparison especially to many countries in Europe. More on that soon.

As previously mentioned, picky eating for some children can become significant enough that a child's nutritional status can be compromised and growth can be inhibited.[15,16] The most recent compilation of official psychiatric diagnoses, the *Diagnostic and Statistical Manual of Psychiatric and Mental Disorders*, fifth edition, now includes a new term called *avoidant and restrictive food intake disorder* to describe some of these kids,[17] listed in the same group as more well-known eating disorders such as anorexia nervosa and bulimia. The emphasis in this chapter will be on children whose fussy eating is problematic but not significantly impacting their growth charts. This is not to say that the research and techniques described here are irrelevant in more extreme situations, but parents of children who meet avoidant and restrictive food intake disorder criteria are certainly encouraged to consult a medical professional who is in a position to offer truly individualized guidance based on a child's particular circumstances.

Noah, who is 5 years old, has never been a strong eater, but more recently he has been able to articulate that one challenge he has when eating is that he is very anxious about vomiting. Noah also has a number of rituals involving counting and touching things in particular ways, and his pediatrician is beginning to wonder if he might meet criteria for obsessive-compulsive disorder. The doctor and Noah's parents are getting increasingly concerned about Noah's behavior as he is not gaining weight as expected for children his age.

## Battlers, Cajolers, and Cavers

It's probably fair to say that most parents of finicky eaters have found themselves belonging to one of three categories. Membership certainly can shift from one category to another on a month-to-month or maybe even meal-to-meal basis, and hybrid approaches are also common. From clinical and personal experience as well as a lot of time spent reading the experiences of others, however, these three groups seem to capture a lot the variance out there, at least when it comes to American parents.

1. *Battlers.* This more traditional approach captured in *A Christmas Story* and many other movies and television shows reflects the glory days of authoritarian parenting and still remains a popular choice, especially among the old school–type parents described in chapter 3. These parents understand the importance of good nutrition and want their children to eat right. A single meal is served to the whole family gathered around the dinner table, and children are expected to eat what is in front of them. If resistance occurs, arguing, shaming, and criticizing soon follow. In more extreme cases, children may be told to sit at the table indefinitely or face other potential punishments until these kids are broken like wild horses and learn to clean their plate without fuss.

2. *Cajolers.* Parents in this category are also concerned about their kids eating a healthy and balanced diet but do everything they can to keep things *positive* as much as possible. Often gathering advice online, these parents will try many of the recommended initiatives that seem to work well specifically with children of bloggers, such as improving child eating habits through getting kids involved in the buying, cooking, and even growing of healthy food. This bounty can then be contorted into colorful works of art, breaded into oblivion, or smothered with ketchup or other kid-friendly condiments. Among this parenting crowd, desserts also tend to be plentiful and used for maximum leverage. Yelling and threatening is kept at a bare minimum, although typically spills out from time to time out of pure frustration and fatigue.

3. *Cavers.* While it would be unfair to say that these parents don't care about their kid's nutrition, the general sentiment for those in this category is

that it just isn't worth the battle to get kids to eat according to those fancy food pyramids you see everywhere. As a result, these children get served their preferred foods, which often involve microwave ovens and take-out containers. Perhaps due to there being less of an investment in food preparation, mealtimes are pretty casual with regard to things like requiring all members of the family to sit together at a single table, turning off televisions, or keeping phones out of reach. These parents often successfully avoid a lot of conflict over meals at home but can really struggle with their kids any place that mac and cheese or chicken nuggets are not immediately available.

These different approaches reflect varying perspectives on parental authority, how kids think, and food itself. For the battlers, there is at least some tacit acknowledgment that things like vegetables just aren't as intrinsically appealing to kids and thus need some extra "encouragement" to get consumed until taste buds mature or a child realizes that it is a lot easier just to eat those lima beans in four quick bites than to spend the rest of the evening parked at the dining room table. In a very developmental or at least sequential way of thinking, this method includes the idea that, over time, these external pressures to eat healthy become unnecessary as a growing child begins to increasingly appreciate the inherent value of healthy food.

For the cajoler group, conflict over food is often interpreted as being less about food and more about power. The idea here is that, as infants turn to toddlers, they are beginning to appreciate that they are distinct beings with desires and goals that are often, maybe too often, different from other people in the world. Baby wants to stay home and play with a toy, but Mommy wants to go to the supermarket. Baby wants to climb the stairs, pull the ears off the dog, and stick her fingers in electrical outlets, but Mommy doesn't think those are such great ideas and *blocks* them from happening. And because Mommy is bigger and better organized, baby doesn't have much control over the outcome.

But not about everything. Baby does have an ace in the hole, and this is where eating comes in. No one, not even Mommy, can make baby eat what she doesn't want to eat. Mommy can make baby's favorite meal, serve it at the perfect temperature, and even play choo-choo or airplane games to get the food playfully near her mouth, but when it comes to actually *eating* it—that's up to baby. And after baby suffers one loss after another in other venues, eating becomes the last stronghold of individual freedom and something not to be given up easily.

It is in this way that mealtimes are hypothesized to reflect a young child's overall desire for autonomy and agency. Knowing this, a parent is better off not furthering the power struggle but rather finding ways around it—hence, the many strategies all designed to convince children that they actually *want* to try that food they have been avoiding for months. This model also suggests that reducing negative interactions and power struggles between child and parents in general could well translate to a reduction in the need for any shows of force around the dinner table.

Cavers see the value in "choosing your battles," which usually does *not* include struggles over food. For many parents in this group, however, this approach is more a practical concession to reality rather than a deliberate approach to mold child behavior. Parents are busy, children are growing—so what's the point of introducing more drama into a family that has plenty without the food battles?

## The Calvary Arrives

These tried and true modes of operation, however, have lately been challenged as some fresh strategies have gained notoriety. From an American perspective, some of these "new" ideas have come from parents who have spent time overseas and have noticed what at least appears to be a much lower prevalence of picky eating in places like France and other European countries. While American kids are whining over the requirement to eat two carrot sticks before being allowed to have dessert, people have noticed that little kids in France are delightfully gobbling down escargot and beet salad. In Karen Le Billon's 2012 book *French Kids Eat Everything*,[18] she notes the positive transformation in her children's eating habits when the family moved from the United States to France and attributes this shift to a number of important differences between the way American and French parents feed their children and approach food in general. These difference include less snacking for European children and a general expectation that a more diverse palate can be learned with experience and routine rather than assuming that children need bland and sweetened foods until some magical day that they don't.

New techniques have also come from experts such as dietitian and family therapist Ellyn Satter, who is widely credited as one of the leaders in the modern approach to picky eating. In articles as well as books such as *Secrets of Feeding a Healthy Family*, she outlines a number of steps that parents can take to make meal times more peaceful and more productive, based on many decades of experience.[19,20] These recommendations, which are embedded in models called the Satter Feeding Dynamics Model and Satter Eating Competence Model[21] describe an important division of responsibility in the family in which *parents are in charge of deciding when the family eats and what foods are served* while *children are left in charge of which foods and how much of them are eaten*. Included in these recommendations is the need for parents to back off from the nagging, bribing, and threatening that occurs at the table. Dessert, for example, is not to be used as an incentive for eating other foods and can even be consumed *first* on days dessert is served at all. Satter also is a firm believer in preparing a single meal for everyone in the family who gather together at a table free of distracting influences like televisions and phones. While not against making certain foods more palatable for children through the use of salt, sauces, and breading, she maintains that her methods will help children grow into "competent" eaters who learn to enjoy food while paying attention to their own internal cues of hunger and satiety. Along the way, she reassures us that the vast majority of children will grow and develop normally with this approach, even if they aren't getting a full serving of fruits and vegetables with every meal. You may have to put zucchini or mashed potatoes on your kid's plate 20 times before it gets eaten, but eventually it *will* get eaten. Overall, this mix of providing structured family meals while not engaging in harsh battles over how much is eaten is described as the authoritative parenting approach to eating.

The critical thinking behind some of these newer strategies comes from the idea that more traditional "clean your plate" methods rob a child of her innate tendency to appreciate the tastiness of healthy food. Logically, the idea here is that the old rewards and punishment model is doomed to fail because the ever suspicious toddler senses that a parent *wants* her to eat those vegetables and thus assumes that anything a parent is pushing that hard *must* be gross and terrible. Resistance then inevitably ensues and quickly a food hierarchy is created in which a treasured dessert can only be had through eating those disgusting healthy foods. By giving a brownie and broccoli equal standing in putting them on the same plate at the same time, a child hopefully comes to recognize that healthy foods are not some obstacle to overcome on the path to a delicious treat but rather yummy options to be enjoyed and savored for their own intrinsic value.

Another critique of traditional food-encouraging methods is that it teaches a child that food consumption should have little to nothing to do with the experience of hunger or satiety and is instead a matter of eating what is in front of you regardless of any internal signals. Children who learn this lesson can then be set up for problems like obesity as their eating behavior becomes increasingly uncoupled to feelings of hunger and more aligned to portion sizes determined by the time of day, wishes of parents, or the volume of a particular food container.[22]

The Satter method and "European" approach, to the degree that each can be seen as single entities, have a number of areas of convergence but do differ in some meaningful ways. Both models emphasize family meals and limiting the grazing of snack foods on demand. At the same time, it is probably fair to say that the Satter methods allow children some additional flexibility with regard to what is eaten and allow parents additional flexibility with regard to what is served than the somewhat more directive European approach. And although my time in France has been limited, it is hard to imagine a dessert being served ahead of its proper place among the courses.

There are also some other approaches out there that share common elements with the Satter and European methods but then deviate on some of the specifics.

For example, one suggestion from sociologist Dina Rose in her book *It's Not About the Broccoli*[23] is to push kids to try new foods but allow them to smell and lick it first and even spit it out if they don't like it. Such a practice is not particularly customary in European families and also runs somewhat counter to Satter's emphasis of not putting pressure on kids to eat. All said, Box 8.1 attempts to consolidate some of the common themes and recommendations put forth by many experts today as well as clarifying where different points of divergence arise.

Many of these suggestions sound relatively easy and may even appear like a welcome relief, but putting them into place can be a challenge, especially for a child who is used to having things done a certain way already. Having permission *not* to nag your kid about eating sounds like a gift from heaven, but for many parents (including me), a physical gag might be required to pull it off. Then there are the looks of betrayal from other parents when you allow your kid to eat the cookie *before* the sandwich at lunch, causing the rest of the crowd to want to follow suit. It also can be tempting simply to mix and match different methods from different programs, but this may compromise some of the major principles that a particular approach is trying to follow. In trying to gain some clarity among all the books and the blogs regarding which particular method is best for your child, we now turn to the recommendations put forth by major professional organizations and the research, or lack thereof, on which these positions are based.

---

### Box 8.1  Expert Suggestions for Fussy Eaters

- Sex: the classification of someone (usually male or female) at birth based on one's external anatomy
- Gender identity: an individual's internal sense of being male, female or somewhere in the middle
- Gender expression: the manifestations of one's gender through things like clothing, language, mannerisms, and preferences
- Sexual orientation: this describes the gender of a person's romantic or sexual attraction
- Trans or transgender: Someone who's gender identity and/or expression does not match their assigned sex
- Gender dysphoria: a feeling of discomfort, anxiety, or even anger about one's assigned sex at birth
- Cisgender: An individual whose gender identity matches their assigned sex
- Gender non-conforming, Non Binary, Genderqueer: A more general term to describe people whose gender expression and identity do not fit traditional distinctions.
- Gender fluid: A dynamic state in which a person's gender identity fluctuates over time

## What the Professional Groups Say

Unlike some of the other topics in this book, like infant co-sleeping or corporeal punishment, the major child development societies don't spend much money on public health announcements for parents of picky eaters. Sure, there is strong support for children eating well, just less airtime on *how,* exactly, to accomplish this feat. Policymakers from the American Heart Association appear to have read Satter's books and recommend an approach of structured family meals without pressure and giving even younger children the responsibility "for whether he or she wants to eat and how much."[24] The American Academy of Pediatrics also seems to have received the same memo in advocating that "it's a parent's responsibility to provide food, and the child's decision to eat it."[25] As part of the Picky Eaters Project, the American Academy of Pediatrics publishes a book of the same name with more specific guidelines and recipes.[26] Similarly, the Academy of Nutrition and Dietetics advises against the use of parental pressure to get children to eat and encourages methods that help children learn to regulate their own food intake.[27] They specifically mention and reference Satter's "division of responsibility" approach as a reasonable model, although note the need for more direct scientific evidence—the topic we turn to next.

## Show Me the Data

Scientists love to say that their chosen area of interest doesn't get the research attention that it should. Picky eating is no different in this regard, but here, it really seems to be true. There just is not that much out there. And what is particularly odd, in my view, is that this relative lack of systematic research exists even though the logistics of conducting good-quality studies on this topic seems much less daunting compared to some other areas covered in the book. In contrast to parenting controversies such as spanking or sleep training where it would be very difficult to find parents willing to be randomized into one group or another, oodles of families would be knocking down the door to participate in a clinical trial in which they are taught and supported to try some specific techniques for a while and then assessed as to the degree that they were effective in areas such as (i) level of conflict at mealtimes, (ii) weight gain, and (iii) status of nutritional parameters like micronutrient levels that might be deficient in some kids. This criticism isn't meant to trash (completely) the value of clinical experience when it comes to helping picky eaters or any other parenting challenge but to acknowledge that this lack of "higher" levels of scientific evidence in this particular area is puzzling.

For whatever reason, then, we need to work with a modest number of smaller studies that often nibble (no pun intended) around the edges of some broader approach but don't tackle the whole thing. In one very small study of mothers of 2- to 5-year-old children who were not necessarily deemed picky eaters, moms were taught the basic principles of something called the Feeding Dynamic Intervention, which was based, perhaps too loosely, on Satter's techniques.[28] The researchers found that the methods were teachable and that there seemed to be a drop in more controlling and restrictive eating behaviors, but there was no control group and no examination of any nutritional parameters in the study. In a published reply to this study, Satter herself notes some points of diversion between the program used in this study and her approach and writes (as of 2015) that "my colleagues and I will be in a position to contribute our own clinical trials to literature."[29p280] In the meantime, some folks seem to be getting a little impatient. In the previously mentioned official position paper about nutrition and children, the American Dietetic Association writes, "In theory, this (Satter's) approach facilitates child self-regulation, but there is no direct evidence to support this approach. The method is, however, consistent with other feeding practices that support healthful eating in children."[27p610]

George H. W. Bush once famously remarked that he never liked broccoli but was forced to eat it as a child. Finally, as president of the United States, Bush declared that he felt that he was finally in a position to say that he never wanted to see broccoli on his plate again.[29] A 2017 review of experimental studies designed to change child eating behavior supported the president's plight and concluded that pressuring kids to eat certain foods while restricting access to favorites tends to be ineffective.[30] It is worth noting here, however, that "pressure," as defined in a research study, is probably much lighter than what often occurs in a child's home. In one of these studies, the coercion used to try to get kids to eat squash soup consisted of a research assistant politely saying, "Finish your soup, please" up to four times.[31] The review further found evidence "that food-based rewards should not be used in order to make children eat every-day, well-accepted foods."[30p329] as this tends to make the nonpreferred food seem even less desirable while elevating the status of the reward food. Modeling also appears to be an important factor in a child's eating habits, although this can work in both directions. Once the most popular and charismatic preschooler in the class declares that she no longer likes apples anymore, you've got a steep hill to climb.

Of course, the studies do not all fall in line with each other. One experiment with teachers and preschoolers tested four different methods of encouraging kids to try new fruits and vegetables: (i) verbally insisting them to try one bite, (ii) inviting them to try the food, (iii) watching others try it (modeling), and (iv) offering a dessert reward, all against a control condition of simply having the food available. The study found that the insisting, rewarding, and inviting all were superior to either modeling or simply having the food available in this short-term study.[32] As many parents also know, following the direction of a parent and following the direction of a teacher can often be two very different things.

The 2017 review also looked at popular initiatives such as cooking programs, school gardens, pairing new foods with old favorites, and giving taste lessons (which, in France, is called the Sapere method). These methods showed some modest benefits, although many of these ideas are designed to help kids in other areas than just eating. Some gains were also found for subtle little tricks or presentations, dryly referred to as "choice architecture" or "nudges" that can make healthy foods more salient and appealing. One study, for example, found that kids ate more carrots on days they were labeled "X-ray vision carrots" (we'll leave legal questions about false advertising aside for now).[33] When it comes to a child playing with their food before eating it, one study did show that allowing preschoolers to do this did increase their consumption of fruits and vegetables, although I'm not sure food playing will ever be a big hit in France.[34]

Altogether, there is a decent but not overly impressive amount of scientific evidence to suggest that the conventional methods through which many parents encourage their kids to eat well, namely nagging, restricting, and rewarding, can often backfire. In its place, many experts now recommend a strategy in which parents provide a solid structure around meals but back off from all the antics to get particular amounts of particular foods in their child's mouth. Research also suggests that these efforts might be easier by also doing things like limiting snacks and engaging children around the growing, preparation, and exploration of good food. For parents of picky eaters who have grown tired of the dreaded mealtime dramas, these suggestions offer some genuine alternatives that are backed by at least some degree of scientific data. That said, there remains a lack of rigorous testing when it comes to showing more definitively that any particular program or technique really works.

Ellie's parents decide to change course and give the Satter method a go. Snacking on demand is eliminated, and the parents decide as a first step to prepare a single dinner for the whole family that can appeal to everyone. Ellie will choose whether or not to eat it and on the 3 days a week there is a dessert, it will be placed with the rest of the meal. The parents explain the new rules to Ellie who looks a little confused. On the first night, Ellie's mother prepares chicken and rice with a side of broccoli. Ellie is also given a cookie. Ellie devours the cookie first and then picks slowly at a little chicken and rice while ignoring the broccoli entirely. Soon thereafter she announces that she's "done." Her parents use all of their willpower to hold their tongues. On subsequent meals, the parents notice some incremental progress in her willingness to try healthier foods and enjoy the much reduced level of acrimony. Ellie definitely seems to be hungrier when it is time for a meal, but improvement is slow and vegetable consumption still meager. She's growing, however, and on the whole the parents are happy with the change in approach.

## It Depends

These general guidelines for picky eating stand to help a lot of families who struggle around mealtimes, but parents can expect that many of them will need to be tweaked and modified based on the individual characteristics of the child. Some trial and error will often be necessary. To help parents find at least a good place to start, here are some adjustments to consider related to specific types of kids.

## Children on the Autism Spectrum

Like pretty much all behaviors, picky eating is determined by a combination of genetic and environmental influences. While the importance of learned behaviors, including exposure to different foods during infancy, can play a significant role in future eating behavior,[35] studies also demonstrate the influence of particular genes such as those involved in chemosensory perception.[36] Highly restrictive eating is also known to be particularly common and particularly intense in some genetically influenced conditions such as autism[37] as well as with various types of emotional-behavioral problems like anxiety disorders.[38] For these kids, a parent may need to incentivize the eating of certain healthy foods to obtain a change in behavior. Yes, this might come at the expense of your child viewing healthy foods as less intrinsically appetizing, but if the Satter-type methods aren't producing results, it's worth a try. Parents may also need to resign themselves to their child's eating habits a bit more in the absence of evidence for any real nutritional deficiency.

For some children with autism or other developmental delays, feeding problems can stem from poor oral muscle tone, gastrointestinal problems, or other causes, necessitating a more rigorous medical and perhaps occupational therapy evaluation. Yet even for younger children with autistic spectrum disorders for whom these problems are not the issue, restrictive eating can remain very challenging. To help, a number of programs have been developed such as the Autism MEAL Plan and the Behavioral Parent Training for Feeding Problems.[39,40] Another approach for somewhat older kids is the Building Up

Food Flexibility and Exposure Treatment (BUFFET) program.[41] These programs involve children and parents working with behavioral specialists for many weeks. The principles underlying these approaches have some consistency with the recommendations proposed by Satter and others with regard to structured meal times and avoiding outright power struggles over food. There are also, however, some important differences. For example, these programs often include actively rewarding children who try new foods with "BUFFET bucks" or other incentives: a general no-no in the more modern feeding recommendations that would see these techniques as too much interference and micromanaging. There is also much more tolerance and even encouragement of children touching, licking, and smelling food than would be permitted in the "European" model.

Do these approaches work? To a degree, the research suggests. The word *help* might be more appropriate than *work*, with what limited studies there are often showing that parents are less stressed out and generally satisfied with the gains that they see, even if the improvement is far from dramatic.[40] These limitations aside, the research suggests that certain children may benefit from a parenting approach that is somewhat more "hands-on" and directive than what is contained in the standard recommendations.

Noah's parents decide to get some help. With their pediatrician's assistance, they get a developmental evaluation for Noah, which concludes that not only does he meet criteria for obsessive-compulsive disorder, he also meets criteria for an autistic spectrum disorder. No specific medical cause for his restrictive eating is found, and the family begins working with a dietician and a psychologist. As Noah's level of anxiety over vomiting slowly comes down, the quantity of food he eats improves, although the acceptable choices remain small. The dietician recommends incentivizing some nonpreferred foods with some prizes he can earn while choosing new foods that don't overly challenge Noah's sensitivities to texture and smell. Over time, Noah's weight stabilizes, and the parents are much less stressed, although they continue to need to make foods specific for Noah and, at least for now, have put aside the dream of the whole family eating the same nutritious meal together.

## Child Temperament Considerations

Many parents of very restrictive eaters may be wondering right about now whether or not the modifications just described for kids with fully diagnosed autism or anxiety disorders should apply to children who have some autistic-like traits or high levels of anxiety but not at levels that would qualify for an official diagnosis. The answer here is likely yes. After all, autism is considered to be a "spectrum" condition, meaning that the behaviors characteristic of autism exist dimensionally and can be present at lower levels in large percentages of kids.[42] The same can be said for things like anxiety disorders, which also represent the upper end of an overall continuum. This means that techniques designed to help kids with particular diagnoses may also be useful for those who are somewhat in that direction but not to the same degree. One study that specifically looked at this issue with regard to selective eating sought to find out whether the presence of more "autism-like" features in a typically developing group of college undergraduates predicted higher levels of food neophobia. Sure enough, a positive association was found.[43]

Temperamentally, children with autistic spectrum disorders tend to have a profile that includes high levels of negative affectivity, low levels of extraversion, and low levels of effortful control: a combination most in line with the anxious category as described in chapter 2.[44] Studies of children who don't meet criteria for autism similarly reveal that higher levels of picky eating are associated with higher levels of trait anxiety (i.e., negative emotionality) and lower levels of sensation seeking (a component of extraversion).[45,46] These associations, of course, don't imply the need for an all-out surrender to the child's limited range of foods but perhaps an appreciation that more heavy-handed approaches have higher probabilities of resulting in a very low "foods eaten-to-battles waged" ratio.

Ayden's parents come to appreciate that his picky eating is largely coming from his anxious temperament and is not a deliberate attempt to expose them as bad parents. They try to involve him more in the selection and preparation of meals to increase his comfort level around food. They cut down on snacking and flexibly offer him the vegetable component of his lunch or dinner as an "appetizer" if he wants to eat a little early. They continue to encourage and praise more adventurous eating but work hard not to have this slide into criticism and judgment. After some discussion, the parents decide that they just aren't ready to offer desserts with the meal but also don't dangle the prospect of dessert to Ayden during dinner as much as they used to do. All this seems to be helping incrementally. Ayden even took several bites of his grilled salmon recently after watching his 2-year-old sister help herself to an amazingly large portion.

## Some Concluding Thoughts

To recap, there's been quite a change in thinking over the past several decades regarding the approach to picky eaters. From the classic notion of parents as being the ones who decide and enforce what and how much a child eats, a more modern approach tries to reduce parent–child battles over food by teaching parents to back off on their demands and transfer the task of regulating food intake back to the child. At the same time, one could also say that many of these same experts recall the Normal Rockwell visions of mealtimes in their criticism of the modern "grab and go" style of eating as they advocate for true family meals that bring parents and children together to enjoy good food and good company.

In recognition that changing a child's eating habits is asking for fairly seismic shifts in behavior, a number of more specific techniques and suggestions such as limiting snacks, encouraging the growing, cooking, and sensory exploration of food, and reintroducing new foods many times before giving up are often part of the package. Major professional organizations from pediatrics, psychology, and nutrition to a large degree have toed the line when it comes to their own official recommendations, creating a high degree of consensus in the message being delivered to parents that is only slightly disrupted from authors, often with experiences from other countries, who push for a somewhat more no-nonsense approach to feeding children.

Behind all the tips and techniques being marketed to parents of picky eaters is a research literature that is sufficient to justify many of the founding tenets of this more contemporary approach but surprisingly thin when it comes to real evidence supporting one particular method over another. For example, there are several studies that demonstrate the ineffectiveness of using a more authoritarian style when it comes to fussy eaters, but whether it really is worthwhile to put the dessert out on the plate with the rest of the dinner, cut peanut butter sandwiches into funny shapes, or re-introduce a new food 5, 7, or 15 times, has really not been established very well. An individual expert or particular program might sound quite prescriptive about what exactly a parent should and shouldn't do, but that doesn't mean that the specific approach, let alone each discrete recommendation, has been thoroughly tested.

It's possible that more rigorous data are coming. Furthermore, there are already some studies out there when it comes to specific programs designed for narrower groups of people, like children on the autism spectrum. While this research also needs to develop, what already exists suggests that some of the regular recommendations may need adjustment for particular groups of kids. Programs built for children with autism, for example, adhere to some of the principles found in things like the Satter methods when it comes to avoiding directives and criticism about food, but these programs also utilize more positive reinforcement strategies such as praise and specific rewards for trying new foods than are typically endorsed more generally. Given the dimensionality of things like autistic spectrum behaviors and anxiety, it is certainly logical to think that similar modifications may need to be made for children who tend temperamentally to be more anxious and less adventurous.

I'm hopeful that some of this uncertainty in the research on picky eating solutions will be received by parents as liberating rather than annoyingly vague. In some ways, this topic more than others is calling for parents to be scientific on a more micro level, as in trying different things with your own child and seeing how it goes. Without really convincing data that compel you to push a specific plan, why not do a little experimenting on your own to find out what actually works with *your* kid? If putting the cookie right next to the vegetable helps your preschooler appreciate the subtle deliciousness of Brussel's sprouts (something I learned much later in life), then terrific—go with it. If he devours the brownie first for a week and then complains of being too full to eat anything else, then maybe it's time for a different plan. If holding off on afternoon snacks and then starting dinner with a veggie appetizer is effective (this one worked well with one of our young sons), then great—let it roll.

Along the same lines, many parents may be realistically appraising their ability to do things like completely shutting off the nagging at meals. To you, I say remember that the research being conducted on picky eating is not done with samples of superparents. This means that the parents in these studies who tried but were not perfectly effective at eliminating the occasional critical and intrusive statement about their child's eating also saw measurable, if not miraculous, improvements in their child's behavior. We mortals can probably expect the same. Also keep in mind that time is also usually our friend when it comes to the number of foods kids are willing to try. It may seem impossible in the moment, but with some good strategies and a willingness to be flexible, that same kid willing to go down with the ship over a single bite of asparagus will be scarfing down sushi and curried chicken in just a few short years—or decades.

## It Depends—Pick Eating

### General Summary

The prevailing opinion on picky eating has moved away from more directive approaches and toward a split of responsibility: the parent decides what foods are served and when, while the child is able to control what and how much is eaten without rewards or punishments given by the parent. Snacking should be limited, the same meal should be served to everyone in the family, and new foods need to be introduced early and often multiple times.

| "It Depends" Factors | Adjustments |
| --- | --- |
| Child temperament—anxious | These children may be especially wary of trying new foods and require some additional incentives to do so. Harsher and more punitive approaches may be even more likely to result in conflict and a smaller number of preferred foods in the future. Incentives could help. |
| Children on the autism spectrum | Food restrictions for these children may be particularly intense and entrenched and may not respond to conventional techniques. Assistance with dieticians and other professionals can be helpful. |

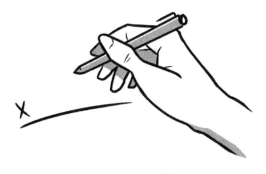

9

# For the Sake of the Kids

## Considerations on Separation and Divorce

This was the chapter I really didn't want to write. Having experienced the separation and divorce of my own parents, only to grow up and put my older two sons through the same thing, this topic was personal. As a result, I questioned my ability to stay sufficiently objective in reviewing the science about the impact of divorce on children and the potential factors that might push those effects in more positive or negative directions. In other words, I was nervous about the answers I might find if I dug too deeply.

When I was 11 years old, my mind was already made up—divorce was a horrible thing to do your kids, especially when a marriage really wasn't *that bad*. There was no domestic violence in my family. In fact, there really wasn't yelling or even spirited arguments (except very occasionally directed at my brother and me). We all got along, lived our lives, and did things together as a family, which was exactly, in my view, how it all was supposed to work. From my perspective, divorce was for couples who had affairs, threw lamps at each other, or had a deadbeat parent who went out and got drunk every night. But since none of those situations seemed to apply, the news of my parents' divorce struck me like a selfish act that put their abstract goals of "being happier" above their commitments to each other (and, more important, to me!). I was mad and let them both know it by telling them their decision was going to "ruin" my life.

But it didn't. There were things I didn't understand about my parents' marriage at the time, and after many ups and downs we all ended up okay. My father starting dating a woman he had known for a while (one of the things I didn't get

Chapter illustrations drawn by Jaq Fagnant

*Parenting Made Complicated.* David C. Rettew, Oxford University Press (2021). © Oxford University Press.
DOI: 10.1093/oso/9780197550977.003.0009

when I was 11), and I saw a happier and more playful side of him emerge. My mother struggled for a while but eventually found someone new herself and is now happily remarried to a thoughtful man who appreciates her in a way my dad never did, or could.

The end result may not have been "happily ever after," but it was hardly the apocalypse that I had originally imagined. Yet despite the softer-than-imagined landing, I swore to myself that divorce was not something I would ever make my own kids endure. Unfortunately, it was, and in 2005, I moved 15 minutes away from my two sons when they were just 3 and 5 years old. My boys were much kinder to me and their mother about this than I had been to my parents, but that didn't stop me from feeling like an utter failure for stepping into a hole that I had been actively trying to avoid my whole life. Once again, however, things turned out well, and both their mother and I were lucky enough to find someone who could bring out the best of us.

The lessons learned and insights gained from these experiences include a better awareness of the bias I now harbor on the subject of divorce. To assuage the guilt that I induced on my parents and to reduce my own culpability for getting divorced myself, I really didn't want to read research studies about how toxic divorce can be for children—much better for my own psyche would be hear that divorce, even in cases when a marriage is not a complete train wreck, does not result in significant harm to children if it is managed skillfully and sensitively. We'll see soon if that indeed is the case.

## In Good Company

Divorce certainly is not an uncommon event. Estimates are that approximately 40% to 50% of first marriages end in divorce,[1] a number that has actually been decreasing for several years.[2] According to the National Center for Family & Marriage Research, divorce rates rose sharply in the 1970s and peaked around 1980 before starting to fall gradually, and then, since 2010, more precipitously to levels now that are near 40-year lows.[3] Yet despite these promising trends, there still are about 1.5 million kids each year in the United States who become children of divorced parents, not to mention parents who separate but were never married in the first place.[4] Of the majority of marriages that remain intact, it is safe to say that many of them struggle too, but the couple remains together for a variety of reasons. For some, this has to do with religious beliefs and the making of a vow for life. For others, there are financial considerations that have to be weighed. And for some couples with children, there is the laudable conviction that the harm that would be caused to the kids from a divorce is too high a price to pay to get out of an unhappy but at least safe and functional marriage.

These parents remain married "for the sake of the kids," at least while the children are young.

> Stephen is a 2-year-old boy whose parents, Gary and Ellen, decided to get married after Ellen became pregnant. Both of them come from religious families and take the vow that they made at their wedding very seriously. To their credit, they've made their marriage work and have learned to enjoy each other's company. At the same time, however, the marriage lacks spark, and both parents secretly concede to themselves that they likely would not have married each other if it weren't for Stephen. This thought has been particularly prominent with Gary lately since he's met a woman through work that seems like a much better fit for him. The thought of being away from Stephen, however, is hard. Stephen is very much attached to both of his parents. He has a cautious and more hesitant nature, and Gary often finds himself in the role of gently pushing Stephen to engage more with his environment.

At the start of the 21st century, well after Western culture had grown accustomed to the idea that lots of marriages ended in divorce or separation and that maybe we shouldn't consider it to be such a big deal, two books, *The Unexpected Legacy of Divorce: A Landmark 25 Year Study*[5] and *The Case for Marriage: Why Married People Are Happier, Healthier, and Better Off Financially*,[6] were published. The first book chronicled in detail a small sample of individuals in California who grew up in divorced households, many of whom grappled a great deal as adults to find love and happiness. In *The Case for Marriage*, a lot of statistics are presented comparing married and nonmarried individuals, most of which converge on the conclusion that with marriage comes a multitude of benefits including longer life, better sex, and bigger wallets. While both books received their fair share of criticism along scientific and political ideology grounds,[7,8] the books provided some uncomfortable challenges to the developing "divorce culture" ready to dismiss divorce as a minor blip in the life of a child.

## How Divorce Might Hurt, or Sometimes Help

Certainly, there are a number of reasons that a divorce could be harmful to kids, and these reasons fall into a number of different categories, as is shown in Figure 9.1.

One of them would relate to more direct psychological effects. These might include heightened feelings of insecurity from having one of the foundational

## How Divorce Can Lead to Negative Effects in Children

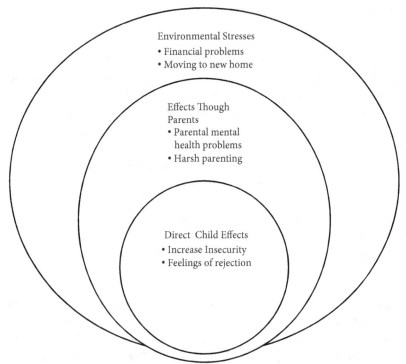

Environmental Stresses
• Financial problems
• Moving to new home

Effects Though
Parents
• Parental mental
  health problems
• Harsh parenting

Direct Child Effects
• Increase Insecurity
• Feelings of rejection

**Figure 9.1** A visual depiction of how divorce can negatively affect children not only though direct child effects but also through impacts on parents and other aspects of a child's larger environment.

pillars of a child's world move away or a sense of rejection that a parent is willing to leave the family. A second category might be described as more practical downstream effects of a divorce such as being the recipient of harsher parenting behavior from a single parent who no longer has anyone to "tag" when feeling overwhelmed or the development of parental mental health problems like depression or substance use, which end up affecting the child. Finally a third group of consequences could be described as broader sociological consequences—many of which can stem from a loss of financial security. There could be the need to move out of one's home or no longer being able to afford some of the enrichment activities a child might otherwise do to help promote healthy development. Indeed, divorce is counted as an official adverse child experience factor, weighted just as heavily as things like parental incarceration or sexual abuse in terms of their risk value for future mental health problems, medical illnesses, and even premature death.[9,10]

> The parents of 4-year-old Hannah just really don't like each other anymore. The mother finds the father to be unmotivated, insensitive, and not at all grateful for the many things she does. For his part, he finds the mother to be critical, controlling, and manipulative. Despite both parent's expressed desire to keep Hannah out of the marital turbulence, the conflict seems to be seeping into her life nonetheless. When Hannah and her father had a recent disagreement, Hannah accused her father of being "invalidating," a word he had never heard her use before in her life (although he heard it often from Hannah's mother). Hannah's parents wonder what the right next step is for this family before the situation becomes poisonous for everyone.

Yet there also is reason to suspect that, as dire as a divorce may sound on the surface, the actual impact of divorce is much less ominous. Following on the heels of the two books warning parents about the dangers of divorce was *For Better or for Worse* in 2002, written by noted marriage scholars E. Mavis Hetherington and John Kelly.[11] Armed with her own long-term sample, the authors countered many of the grim conclusions reached by others in finding that the negative consequences for children are hardly inevitable and that some children may even become better able at managing stress through the navigation of their parents divorce.

Often missing in discussions about the negative effects of divorce is a consideration of the alternative. In other words, what happens to children when their parents stay in an unhappy but intact marriage? After all, parents do not generally end perfectly good relationships, and this fact makes simple comparisons between children of divorced parents and children in intact families a bit unfair. A methodologically better but more difficult comparison sample to collect for a research study would be children whose parents are not particularly satisfied with the marriage but choose to stay together anyway. From this perspective, it's not difficult to imagine that there may be instances in which an unhappy couple who stays together could result in higher levels of problems for kids. There could be high levels of open conflict and even domestic violence that a child is forced to witness on a regular basis. There could be parental disengagement from the family that, for all intents and purposes, feels like a rejection to a child. And, of course, there can be the child's exposure to all the reasons why the marriage isn't working in the first place.

Five-year-old Brittany has already seen too much. Her parents, who have never been married, are in constant conflict, and Brittany's originally sweet and curious temperament has shifted over the past year to being more angry and reactive. Brittany's father drinks, which causes him to be nasty and, at times, abusive. Her mother has become increasingly concerned about their safety but is also worried about how they would make ends meet on their own.

Given all the different factors and scenarios that can lead to perfectly logical claims that divorce is a major disaster in the life of a child, a welcome relief from ongoing strife, or something in between, we once again have to plunge into the data and discover what really has been found on this important subject.

## Researching the Effects of Divorce on Children

Simple comparisons looking at the long-term outlook for kids who have grown up in divorced versus intact families reveals a number of worrisome associations, with children from divorced families having higher rates of mental health problems, substance abuse, teen pregnancy, and educational underachievement.[12] In the immediate period following a divorce, it is common for children to exhibit a number of negative emotions and behaviors including anger and defiance, withdrawal, sadness, anxiety, and increased need for attention.[11] Over the long term, however, it has been estimated that 75% of children will *not* have sustained problems after about 2 years post-divorce (unless there continue to be significant ongoing stressors), and that the magnitude of the troubles that do continue are often rather small.[1,13,14] As one expert puts it, "research supports the view that the long-term outcome of divorce for the majority of children is resiliency rather than dysfunction."[15p.968] There is also evidence, however, that children from divorced parents will have higher divorce rates themselves as adults, in part due to a view of marriage as something other than a lifelong committment.[5,13]

Looking across a number of indicators of adjustment including different types of child behavioral problems, academic achievement, and relationship quality, a meta-analysis by psychologist Paul Amato in 2001 found stronger links between divorce and child behavioral problems than with academic performance.[16] One caveat, however, was that the more scientifically rigorous the study was, the weaker the association between divorce and mental health got.[16] In terms of the magnitude of these difference, Amato calculated that if all of the differences between children of divorced versus intact families were actually due to the divorce itself (a really big *if*), divorce leads to 1 in 10 individuals having more mental health problems, 1 in 5 individuals having higher levels of discord in their own marriage, and 1 in 3 individuals having a poorer father–child relationship.[8] These are certainly not trivial amounts, but less than many of the more catastrophic conclusions that have been made in the past.[17]

What makes many experts skeptical about drawing conclusions from studies that simply compare nonrandomized subjects who have and have not experienced a parental divorce is the strong likelihood that what might easily appear as an effect of the divorce itself is actually due to other things. Many of these factors will be soon discussed in the "It Depends" section. With divorce, as in many parent-related topics, one nagging issue is genetics and the possibility that there are inherited tendencies that put people at risk for *both* divorce and mental health problems like depression or substance use. Perhaps surprising to some, there does appear to be genetic influences on the likelihood of getting a divorce, and these may be related to the inheritance of certain personality traits, particularly low extraversion, high negative emotionality, and low effortful control (using the terms described in chapter 2).[18] Sorting these different influences out can involve some interesting research maneuvers, such as using twins or children who have been adopted. One study compared biological versus adopted children after a divorce and found that both groups showed post-divorce increases in mental health struggles, suggesting that the parental divorce itself was playing a role. In contrast, problems with social functioning and school achievement were present only in the biological children, indicating that these changes may actually reflect an underlying genetic effect masquerading as a direct result of the divorce.[19] Of course, a different study that examined children from identical versus fraternal twins found a different pattern.[20] These varying results can be confusing, but the bottom line here is that, if you don't look carefully, it can be easy to attribute child difficulties coming from other sources as being all due the divorce itself.

## It Depends

With these broad conclusions and their limitations in mind, it is time to move to the considerable number of "it depends" factors that have been demonstrated to be important when it comes to the emotional, behavioral, and cognitive effects of divorce on children. As Hetherington notes quite well, "it is not the inevitability of divorce outcomes, but the diversity of outcomes following divorce that is striking."[21p.164] This diversity comes from the large number of variables that can spell the difference between one child experiencing a very rocky road after a divorce and another who rapidly is able to get back on his feet.

# Age

While it's not hard to imagine that a child's age could have something to do with his adjustment to a parental divorce, predicting whether an older age would be protective or put the child at additional risk is a lot more challenging. On the one hand, you might think that older children would be better off, as they usually have more emotional regulation skills than the little ones, and, from a cognitive standpoint, they also tend to have a more developed sense of perspective of what is and isn't happening. But that cognitive skill could also be a liability, because older kids really *get* what is going on and what it means, while younger children may not fully appreciate the situation. Younger kids also can be a little more flexible with regard to things like moving back and forth between households. From my own experience, I always marveled how my own sons, even at older ages, could just in a matter-of-fact way ask whether they were sleeping at my house or their mother's that night and be fine with it. If I didn't know where *I* was sleeping on any given night, I would be a lot grouchier.

Given these different theories, it is maybe not surprising that the research on this topic is mixed and complex. Even this "it depends" factor has some "it depends" thrown in the mix. One study, for example, found that a divorce that occurred when children were in elementary school had more associations with later behavioral problems in comparison to kids of middle school age. However, when it came to academic grades, the pattern was reversed.[22] In another study that followed a group of American children from before kindergarten to the 10th grade, divorce that occurred, for boys, during the elementary school years was related to increased and persistent aggressive and defiant behaviors. In contrast, a divorce that occurred when the boys were in middle school was associated with a temporary bump in these behaviors, which then dropped after 1 year and actually then fell below baseline levels.[23] The authors commented that this may perhaps be due to the boys responding positively to having lower levels of conflict in the house.

Overall, based on some research that is fairly old by now and probably in need of attention once again, the weight of evidence seems to suggest that preschool and elementary school-aged children may have the most trouble coping with a parental divorce compared to older children.[24,25] On the flip side, however, some of these same studies suggest that younger children may also be more likely to accept a parent having a new partner or spouse. Practically speaking, parents are usually not in a position to flexibly *time* their separation anyway, but it can be useful to consider how age can fall into the equation here. A separation, for example, that will involve a child needing to move to another town might be especially tough for older children but not so bad for younger ones. On the other hand, being a single parent could be proportionally more taxing for someone with young children given the amount of adult time these kids usually need.

## Gender

There has been some evidence that girls from divorced household are more likely than boys to experience the extreme of either a very negative or positive outcome later in life. One the one hand, research indicates that these girls are more at risk for not completing either high school or college.[21] This, in turn, can lead to financial hardships in adulthood, especially if she winds up being a mother herself earlier in life. On the other hand, some of the same researchers have also found that girls may also be very resilient after a parental divorce and become very high-achieving and successful adults. Overall, it is probably fair to say that gender differences when it comes to adjustment after a divorce have not been found to be particularly *prominent* "it depends" factors, especially compared to some of the other ones to be addressed next.[26,27] They are also not something that you generally are going to be able to affect anyway as a parent (see chapter 7), so we'll move on.

## Mental Health and Child Temperament

A cardinal finding when it comes to studying the effects of difficult experiences on people is that *one the best predictors of how well someone will fare after a stressful event is how well the person was faring before the stressful event.* The effect of divorce on children seems to be no different with research showing that children who had adjustment problems prior to a divorce had higher levels of adjustment problems after the separation.[28] This observation does not mean, however, that these kids necessarily took a bigger emotional "hit" from the actual divorce.[29] Among other things, there instead may be a role of genetics, with similar genes in both a parent and child contributing to mental health problems and relationship difficulties, or it could reflect that fact that serious marital problems have already exerted a negative effect on child behavior even before parents decide to go their own ways.

Translating all of this into more temperamental terms, we might predict that those with more challenging temperaments, such as those in the agitated group, may be at higher risk of struggling behaviorally after something like a divorce in comparison to kids who have temperaments that traditionally have been called "easy" (encompassing the mellow or even the moderate group).[24] A couple of studies have looked directly at this question.[30,31] In one study of children between 9 and 12 years of age,[31] overall level of adjustment post-divorce was found to be related to a child's feeling of rejection, but this was true primarily for kids who were low in positive emotionality, a trait similar to extraversion and surgency described in chapter 2. More inconsistent parenting was also found to be related to adjustment, particularly among kids who were more impulsive temperamentally (a component of higher negative emotionality and lower effortful control). In a larger study of younger children ranging between 1 and 10 years old who were then followed for up to 8 years, those from divorced families who went on to develop high levels of oppositional and defiant behavior tended to be the ones who had problems originally. Overall, these findings suggest that child temperament dimensions are interacting with aspects of parenting practices and other variables to shape how well kids cope after a divorce.

What should you do with this information if you are considering or in the process of separation and have a child who is temperamentally vulnerable to stress? For those on the fence about splitting up, this could be a motivating factor to double down on efforts to try to improve the relationship first. If divorce is a foregone conclusion, parents may want to have a low threshold in getting some help in the way of counseling and psychotherapy for the child to try to minimize the negative impact. Consideration could also be given to separation arrangements that minimize disruption to the child, such as "birdnesting" which allows the child to remain at the family home while the parents take turns being there with the child.

> Stephen's parents predict that he would have a very difficult time with a divorce and decide to redouble their efforts to make their marriage work. They look to their faith for strength and support and begin working with a marriage counselor. After 6 months, there is noticeable improvement, although their marriage remains far from ideal. Stephen's parents take a hard look at the big picture and decide, at least for now, that things are "good enough."

## Parenting Quality

Theoretically, this "it depends" factor could really tilt the impact of divorce in significant ways. If the person who leaves the home was one whose parenting style was particularly problematic, a divorce could be expected to benefit a child through the improved parenting quality a child receives. On the other hand, a divorce itself could lead to more negative parenting practices as the remaining parent or parents struggle to do everything on their own without a partner to step in when that person is starting to run out of gas. There are also just fewer people around to help supervise kids and keep them out of trouble.[32]

There are data to suggest that higher-quality parenting after a divorce can reduce its negative impact.[33,34] As for overall parenting quality getting worse post-separation, that phenomenon has been more difficult to document, as research suggests that at least some of the negative parenting, often interpreted as a *consequence* of the divorce, was present many years earlier.[35] A meta-analysis by Amato that focused on noncustodial fathers found that while the absolute amount of contact did not relate to how well children were doing after a divorce, having a closer bond and using a more authoritative parenting style was associated with the children having more academic success and less emotional-behavioral problems.[36] A similar result was found in a study that focused on mothers.[37]

These findings suggest that being able to maintain your "A game" as a parent can be very beneficial to your child after a divorce. Staying warm, having positive interactions, minimizing harsh and critical comments—all of these things make a difference in a child's adjustment. But as someone who's been there, this is much easier said than done. To pull it off, parents need to take care of themselves, accept support from others, and actively resist passing the baton of negative thoughts and feelings that inevitably come into our brain on to our kids. Sparing children all the negative thoughts you might have about the *other* parent is also paramount. Those thoughts might be entirely valid, but they are better expressed to counselors or friends than kids. Like two nuclear armed countries, parents have the power of mutually assured destruction when it comes to how children view their parents, with the kids becoming the collateral damage.

The supportive but firm family therapist working with Hannah's family tells the parents that, when it comes to using their child as a vessel for their complaints of each other, it was time to "knock it off." After explaining the negative influence of this practice on Hannah, the mother and father agree to find other avenues to vent their frustrations. While continuing in the process of separation, they work toward each of them finding the time and space to have enjoyable experiences with their daughter while maintaining similar limits and rules across both households. Hannah continues to struggle with the divorce, but her anger at both parents changes into feelings of loss and sadness that she can more freely express.

## Parental Conflict

While parental divorce can be hard, many children have already been forced to cope with years of marital conflict. [38] This could include a child having to witness intense arguments between parents, outright domestic violence, or a parent frequently storming out of the house, maybe this time for good. There can also be hostile and irritable interactions between parents and children that often flow downstream of marital battles, in addition to manipulative and more subtle efforts of one parent to pit a child against the other parent to gain favor.

As would be expected, there is convincing evidence that indicates that it is the level of interpersonal conflict between parents that is responsible for many of the associations between divorce and negative child outcomes, rather than the divorce per se.[24] Indeed, some studies indicate that when parental conflict is taken into account, the independent effect of divorce is no longer present at all.[39] An important study by Gloria Moroni from the United Kingdom has further weakened the case that it is the divorce itself that is driving most of the struggles seen in kids.[40] Following a large group of parents and their children from ages 9 months to 12 years, the study found that the differences present with regard to cognitive skills and mental health status between children of divorced versus married parents was largely due to *other* factors. Research has documented this finding in the past, but what was interesting about this study was that it showed that this important other factor was different when it came to children's cognitive status versus their behavior. Specifically, the difference in cognitive ability was very much a function of parental education while being fairly insensitive to levels of family conflict. By contrast, the higher levels of behavioral problems in children of divorced parents were strongly related to the level of parental conflict but not parental education. Amount of financial resources, interestingly, was related to both domains. In trying to interpret what her results mean on a practical basis, she argues that interventions targeting poverty, level of parental conflict, and parental education are likely to be more helpful to the children of divorced parents than efforts to try to reduce divorce itself.

Other work, however, isn't so fast to let parents who might like to escape from unhappy but otherwise stable marriage off the hook so easily. One important investigation prospectively followed a group of parents and their offspring for 12 years as the children moved into young adulthood.[41] Like others, they found that the effect of divorce on a child's overall level of well-being depended a great deal on the level of marital conflict. In making a strong case for divorce among high-conflict couples, the researchers found that when parents from high-conflict marriages divorced, their kids were happier and less distressed compared to kids from high-conflict marriages who parents stayed together. Indeed, these offspring from divorced high-conflict parents were doing about as well as offspring from low-conflict nondivorced families. However, the study also found that offspring from low-conflict families were doing better if their parents stayed together rather than divorced. Surprisingly, in looking at the children of divorced parents as young adults, it was those who came from low-conflict households who were struggling the most. While it is important to note that the parental divorce for children in this study tended to occur in adolescence, the authors hypothesized that the impact of divorce in low-conflict families may have come from them being unprepared for it. They write, "In these cases, the children may react with shock and disbelief, and divorce was likely to represent an unwelcome and uncontrollable long-term decline in quality of life."[41p913]

> Brittany's mother decides to take a major step. One night when the father is out drinking, she takes Brittany out of state to return to her parent's home. A restraining order against the father is filed, and the mother looks to gain custody of Brittany. The father is furious but in the end puts up little legal resistance. Brittany is initially frightened with the abrupt transition but then seems to be able to relax and settle into her safer surroundings.

As described in the example, there may be advantages to having a single custodial parent after a divorce rather than joint custody in marriages that were very high in conflict. The idea here is that if divorced parents are forced into continued interaction with each other, then there will be more arguing and fighting, which will have continuing negative effects on the child. Overall, research suggests that children in joint custody arrangements do *better* with regard to social, academic and mental functioning in comparison to those in sole maternal custody,[42] but this association may not hold for high-conflict families. As people have observed, the perceived advantage of joint custody could reflect other factors that *underlie* the decision to have joint versus sole custody rather than an effect of the custody itself.[1]

## A Mostly Encouraging Message

Overall, the research is quite clear that at least a large part of what might easily look like a negative causal effect of divorce on child mental health and academic performance can be accounted for by other factors, many of which are present prior to the divorce. These include genetic influences, a child's temperament and baseline level of functioning, and amount of parental and family conflict. Some studies suggest that taking these other factors into account makes the direct effect of divorce go away completely,[43] while other studies show that an, albeit smaller, effect of divorce remains.[8,14] Regardless, there is a lot of science that conveys the reassuring message that the majority of children actually weather a divorce quite well, particularly if many of the "it depends" factors are positive such as maintaining good parenting practices and keeping the level of conflict between the parents to a minimum (and keeping the children out of that conflict as much as possible). The subsequent relationships parents make also certainly impact a child's adjustment. Simply replacing one troubled and antagonistic partner for another (and another) is definitely not doing a child any favors. Conversely, those parents who are fortunate enough to find love and greater happiness with someone new are likely to find that some of these positive changes percolate down to the kids as well.

All that said, a parental divorce remains a tough transition for kids and not one to be taken lightly. As described earlier, this might be particularly true for children who didn't see a divorce coming and who weren't subject to high levels of conflict and hostility. This means that a child who is old enough and who has the cognitive capacity to truly understand the change that is coming from a divorce can be expected to voice their unhappiness about it, thereby stomping, intentionally or otherwise, on an open wound of parental guilt. These moments can easily provoke a parent to become defensive and angry or to shift immediately into "fix-it" mode by listing all the *good* things about Mommy and Daddy going their separate ways. Such reactions are quite understandable, but unproductive. As painful as it is, this is one of those times where a parent needs to suck it up and tolerate the idea that they have contributed to at least the temporary distress of their child, who has every right in the book to complain about it.

Coming back to my own personal experience with divorce, I'm left feeling *mostly* good with the way things turned out. As a child of divorced parents, I have subsequently learned about some of the troubles my parents had and was grateful for the gift of ignorance I had at the time. Yet, despite their very real difficulties with each other, the unified message I received as an adolescent was that *both* parents were going to stay in my life, and *both* parents continued to deserve love and respect. I benefited from those beliefs. As a father raising two children who weathered a divorce better than I did, I also have to admit to being the beneficiary of some unpredictable and pretty random circumstances (sorry, destiny believers) that dramatically changed my life and the life of my kids for the better.

## It Depends—Divorce

### General Summary

While there is evidence that parental divorce is associated with a higher likelihood of mental health and academic problems, most children endure a parental divorce with minimal long-term problems. Research indicates that a large proportion of the association between divorce and negative outcomes is accounted for by other factors described here.

| "It Depends" Factor | Adjustment |
| --- | --- |
| Child temperament | More difficult adjustment after a divorce was found among children with low levels of extraversion, high impulsivity, and high negative emotionality, although these traits were often present before the divorce. |
| Parenting quality | An authoritative parenting style after a divorce may help minimize the negative effects. |
| Parental conflict | Children whose parents are in high-conflict marriages may do better after a divorce while those coming from low-conflict marriages can struggle more. Reducing parental conflict can reduce some of the negative effects of divorce. |

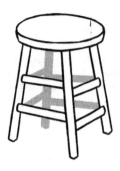

# 10

# Sparing the Rod (and the Chair?)

## Spanking, Time-Outs, and Other Disciplinary Techniques

In the opening of the 1994 film *Wyatt Erp*, which portrays the life of one of the most famous sheriffs of the Old West, a teenage Erp tries to run off in the middle of the night to fight alongside his brothers in the Civil War. His father, played by Gene Hackman, catches him on horseback and brings Wyatt back home. As the two ride together on the same horse with Wyatt's arms wrapped around his father, Hackman calmly discusses his son's disobedience and lets him know gently, almost lovingly, that, "You know, I'm going to have to whip you some." Wyatt merely nods in agreement and thus begins the story of one of America's most iconic symbols of old school justice.

To many, scenes like this depict corporal punishment the way it should be (without the whip, of course): a method of discipline that a parent rationally chooses at an appropriate moment, which results in a child who respects authority and lives honorably within the laws of society. But to increasingly large numbers, corporal punishment is not discipline at all but rather a form of violence that is too often used in the heat of the moment. In their eyes, spanking and other forms of corporal punishment don't reduce the chances of future behavioral problems but rather sets in motion a cycle of aggression that harms the quality of the parent–child relationship and ultimately *increases* the odds that a child will act violently in the future. Even in the movie, it turns out that one of Wyatt's main flaws in the eyes of others is that he too quickly resorts to physical aggression to enforce the law.

Chapter illustrations drawn by Jaq Fagnant

*Parenting Made Complicated*. David C. Rettew, Oxford University Press (2021). © Oxford University Press.
DOI: 10.1093/oso/9780197550977.003.0010

Societies across the world increasingly seem to be turning to this second point of view. In part due to disturbingly high rates of outright child abuse, the cultural tide has begun to turn against corporal punishment, at least with regard to official stances and policy and our new "woke" culture. According to the Global Initiative to End All Corporal Punishment in Children, corporal punishment is now illegal in the home in 53 countries and is illegal in schools in 131 countries as of January 2018.[1] Supporting this stance, a recent study found that the rate of physical fighting among male and female adolescents living in countries in which corporal punishment is illegal is 69% and 42% that of the rate in countries where it is legal, respectively.[2] The list of countries where spanking is illegal is diverse and includes countries like Argentina, the Republic of Congo, Germany, Poland, and South Sudan. The United States is listed as a country "without a clear commitment to law reform." Spanking and corporal punishment remain legal at home in all states (with some stating provisions against "excessive" force or causing bodily harm), although it is unlawful at school in 31 of them. Indeed, some states such as Nevada and Oklahoma have even passed legislation to remind parents that it remains a legitimate option. The Department of Education estimates that in 2016 more than 160,000 children received corporal punishment in a school.[3]

In the 1960s, almost 95% of adults thought spanking and other forms of corporal punishment were an acceptable form of discipline.[4] This level of support has waned over the ensuing decades, although by not nearly as much as many people might have expected.[5] As Figure 10.1 shows, an ongoing national survey from the University of Chicago reveals that support for the statement, "It is

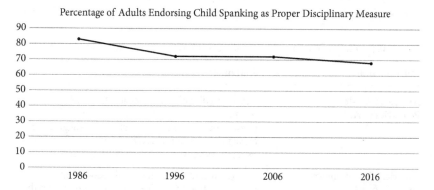

Percentage of Adults Endorsing Child Spanking as Proper Disciplinary Measure

**Figure 10.1** Decreasing endorsement by parents for the statement, "It is sometimes necessary to discipline a child with a good, hard spanking," over time. While this rate has been falling, approval remains high and in the majority. Data from the General Social Survey, University of Chicago.

sometimes necessary to discipline a child with a good, hard spanking" was 83% in 1986, dropping to 72% in 1996 and 2006 and, most recently, remaining in the majority at 68% in 2016.[6]

Indeed, the popular term "a slap on the wrist" continues to be used to denote a punishment that is too *light* or lenient. This continued endorsement for the use of spanking does show some differences related to geography, religious and political affiliations, and ethnicity.[7] Many, of course, also view the option of spanking as a parental, even religious, freedom, looking to the Bible as a source of support for corporal punishment in the oft-quoted line "Spare the rod and spoil the child," from Proverbs 13:24.

> Melissa and Bill aren't sure what to do with their 4-year-old boy Alex. He frequently misbehaves at home and gets into a lot of physical fights with his 7-year-old brother. His preschool teacher has also voiced some concern that Alex can antagonize other children. The parents have different views as to what should happen next. Bill recalls that he was somewhat the same way as a child and that his parents responded by spanking him when he misbehaved. Bill thinks this was helpful and that he "turned out alright." Melissa is hesitant about spanking and wants to ask their pediatrician at their next check-up.

This persistently high level of support for corporal punishment is remarkable given that, over the past 40 years, the official line from nearly all of the prominent professional associations has profoundly moved against spanking as a legitimate disciplinary technique, as summarized in Table 10.1.

A report from 2000 showed that only 4% of psychologists in clinical practice would endorse the use of spanking at a frequency higher than "rarely."[8]

Table 10.1 Official Positions on Spanking from Major Professional Organizations.

| Organization | Statement |
| --- | --- |
| American Academy of Pediatrics (AAP) | "If you feel discipline is necessary, the AAP recommends that you do not spank or use other physical punishments. That only teaches aggressive behavior, and becomes ineffective if used often. Instead, use appropriate time outs for young children."[10] |
| American Psychological Association (APA) | "…the American Psychological Association recognizes that scientific evidence demonstrates the negative effects of physical discipline of children by caregivers and thereby recommends that caregivers use alternative forms of discipline that are associated with more positive outcomes for children."[12] |
| American Academy of Child and Adolescent Psychiatry (AACAP) | "…does not support the use of corporal punishment as a method of behavioral modification."[11] |

The American Academy of Pediatrics, in its discouragement of corporeal punishment, writes that spanking "teaches that causing someone pain is OK if you're frustrated."[9] In December 2018, the AAP published new guidelines advising pediatricians more forcefully that they should council parents "not to use corporal punishment."[10] The American Academy of Child and Adolescent Psychiatry similarly states that it "does not support the use of corporal punishment as a method of behavioral modification."[11] The American Psychological Association, meanwhile, has also issued a relatively new resolution in 2019 that broadly discourages corporal punishment.[12]

Thus, for an increasing number of experts in child development and behavior, the scientific case against spanking has been decidedly made, and there is little basis left to claim that the issue is really even controversial anymore. In fact, many of these folks are so convinced about the negative effects of corporal punishment that they have moved on to scrutinizing "milder" types of punishments such as time-outs, as we will discuss later in this chapter.

Yet all this should not be taken to mean that there don't remain some pediatricians and other child advocates who continue to want to see spanking as a viable option. The American College of Pediatricians, a small group of pediatricians known for more conservative perspectives on many parenting matters, writes in their official position on the subject that "disciplinary spanking by parents, when properly used, can be an effective component in an overall disciplinary plan with children."[13] Their stance is based mainly on their critique of the quality of the scientific literature against spanking that we will cover soon.

Five-year-old Carla comes from a tight-knit family. She is the youngest of four children. During the course of an evaluation for a possible anxiety disorder, Carla reveals that she gets spanked occasionally when she misbehaves and that this happened with her older siblings too. While it is also apparent during the interview that the parents show a lot of warmth and support for their kids, the evaluating clinician focuses on the spanking as a primary source for Carla's anxiety. The parents are a bit taken back by this and explain that they only do this occasionally and are careful not to spank reactively out of anger. They believe their kids accept spanking as an appropriate method of discipline and wonder if they should seek out a second opinion about their child's anxiety.

This growing chasm between persistent public opinion and most expert consensus on the issue of spanking is raising the stakes of this topic politically. As state child protective agencies increasingly view corporal punishment as blurring into child abuse, many parents worry that an overzealous social worker could now swoop in and remove a child from their home for what they would consider a fundamental right of parenting. While few condone the striking of a child with objects or a closed fist, some parents express unease that the line between reasonable corporal punishment and physical abuse is becoming too muddled in the eyes of many state child welfare agencies, causing firm but loving parents to need to look over their shoulders for overreaching and, in their eyes, unnecessary government interference. Many of these same parents see society's growing rejection of spanking and corporal punishment as a major cause behind their perception of a new generation of youth that is increasingly undisciplined and disrespectful.

## What Exactly Is Corporal Punishment?

Before jumping into the research on the effectiveness and long-term effects of spanking and corporal punishment, it's important to define what is and what is not meant by these terms. Putting aside the view of some that corporal punishment is always a form a child maltreatment,[14] the research literature generally puts some parameters on what specifically distinguishes corporal punishment from child abuse. These often include the following elements.[15]

1. An intent to discipline rather than to harm
2. An action that is not severe enough to cause injury
3. Using an open rather than closed hand on the buttocks or other extremities like the wrist
4. Using it only when parents are in control of themselves and not in a fit of rage

When people use the term *spanking*, it is generally meant to convey the hitting of a child specifically on their buttocks, although some definitions include the striking of other body extremities. This boundary, often applied in research studies too, coincides with the line that many parents try to adhere to as well, although certainly there are parents who can slip into doing more extreme forms of physical punishment. Indeed, as we will soon see, it is these folks who engage in "regular" spanking but who will also occasionally strike their child out of anger that complicate a lot of the research on this subject.

## The Scientific Evidence on Spanking

Much of the research on spanking and corporal punishment has focused on two main questions, namely, (i) Does spanking *work* to stop the behavior that a parent is trying to stop? and, perhaps more important, (ii) Does spanking lead to negative outcomes in the future with regard to things like higher levels of child aggression, worse mental health problems, and a poorer parent–child relationship.

At this point, there is quite a bit out there on spanking and enough to satisfy many child behavior experts that definitive conclusions can now be made. From the literally hundreds of studies that now exist on the efficacy and long-term consequences of spanking, efforts to summarize this vast amount of data have been made since the 1960s.[15] There exists enough research that there have been at least five meta-analyses published on spanking that have tried to combine many studies into one large data set.[15-19] While none of them conclude with a ringing endorsement for spanking, the various meta-analyses have come out in different places with regard to *exactly how bad* spanking is for kids, ranging from quite a bit, to a little, to no harm under certain circumstances.

One of the more damning reviews of spanking was written in 2002 by Elizabeth Gershoff who was then at Columbia University.[17] In her review of 88 studies that had been performed to date, she found that while there was modest evidence to support the idea that spanking did result in immediate compliance, it came at the cost of worse outcomes along 10 different areas including higher levels of child aggressive behavior, decreased quality of the parent–child relationship, future criminal and antisocial behavior, and abusing one's own child or partner as an adult. Another meta-analysis published in 2004 found similar results, although the magnitude of the negative behaviors associated with spanking was smaller.[16]

## Debate On

The study by Gershoff received a fair amount of press, with articles in the *New York Times*,[20] CBS News,[21] and other prominent media outlets covering the study and challenging parents to reconsider their disciplinary strategies. Critiques of the study also began to emerge immediately, including a written reply to the study that was published in the same journal edition.[22] This response countered that there were serious problems with the way the analyses were conducted and interpreted. Specific complaints included the fact that many of the studies used for the meta-analysis were cross-sectional (meaning that they measured only one point in time and thus can't distinguish between spanking actually causing problem behavior versus the other way around) and often relied on subjects' retrospective accounts of how they were treated as a child. Perhaps most important, too many of the studies in the review included subjects who not only spanked their kids but did things like hit them with objects or used corporal punishment as the primary mode of discipline. Consequently, negative effects that are really due to parents using very harsh and abusive behavior can appear to be due to properly used spanking in a classic example of throwing out the baby with the bathwater.

One of the authors of this letter, psychologist Robert Larzerele, then followed up with his own meta-analysis, which, not surprisingly, came up with a very different conclusion. This meta-analysis included 26 studies, with only 8 of them being in common with the Gershoff study.[19] Instead of looking just at studies of corporal punishment on its own, Larzerele and his colleagues focused on research that compared corporal punishment to other punishment techniques such as time-outs in an effort to control for the very real possibility that kids requiring frequent parental disciplinary interventions *of any kind* are more likely to be the ones with higher levels of behavioral and other mental health problems. Finally, the authors also divided corporal punishment into whether it was being used conditionally (once in a while after other things have failed), customarily (used more regularly), predominantly, or in more severe forms. What they found was that while spanking that was used in severe forms or as the predominant form of discipline was indeed related to more negative behavior, more conditional use was actually associated with slightly more compliance and less antisocial behavior when compared to other disciplinary techniques.

Around and around we started to go with reviews putting up dueling evidence that seemed to be supporting whatever the primary researcher had been wanting to say all along. To the parents paying attention to these intellectual debates, these mixed messages were confusing and frustrating. Why couldn't science agree, and why did it have to be so complicated? In some ways, it didn't. Everybody knew what needed to happen to perform the definitive study on spanking; it just was impossible to do it as described in chapter 1 regarding what would be involved in doing an actual randomized controlled trial for corporal punishment. As a consequence, we are forced to use less rigorous designs that try to measure what parents are doing with their children already and then apply statistical methods to separate the effects of spanking from all the other potentially important factors (how much positive interactions parents have with their kids, level of child behavior problems before the corporal punishment began, etc.) that may be coming along for the ride.

One place, however, where it might be possible to use a more experimental approach is to look at treatment studies of oppositional and defiant children to see if any improvements in child behavior they achieved worked *through* parents spanking less. While such an analysis in spanking research has not been utilized often, one study using the popular Incredible Years program to help parents of 3- to 8-year-old kids manage defiant and aggressive behavior did indeed find that reductions in spanking appeared to be one of the mechanisms through which the program was effective.[23] It is also worth noting that nearly all of the main evidence-based parenting guidance programs never have or no longer use spanking in their recommended procedures and continue to show positive results in reducing a child's level of negative behaviors.

## New Research Thickens the Plot

Moving into more recently conducted research, a newer stab at summarizing the spanking data was published in 2013 by Ferguson.[18] The wrinkle to this meta-analysis was the attempt to extract "pure" spanking from a broader array of more intense kinds of physical punishment. The bottom line from this investigation was that *both* spanking and more broadly defined physical punishment were significantly related to negative behavior and poorer cognitive performance, although the magnitude of these associations were considered strong for more broadly defined physical punishment while being small for more narrowly defined spanking.

In 2016, Gershoff comes back again to offer an updated analysis from her previous effort more than a decade earlier.[3,15] This time around, she and colleague Andrew Grogan-Kaylor really tried to address the criticism leveled against the earlier review by separating spanking from more severe forms of physical punishment in their analyses of the research data. In total, this meta-analysis combined data from over 160,000 children. Overall, the results of their new review decidedly showed that spanking was related to a number of undesirable outcomes such as increased child aggression and delinquent behavior, poorer parent–child relationship, lower self-esteem, increased mental health problems such as depression, and an increased likelihood of being a victim of physical abuse. Looking across all the statistically significant associations that were calculated between spanking and these different outcomes, 99% of them indicated that spanking was linked to negative rather than positive child outcomes. For example, of the 27 studies that looked at the relations between spanking and child aggression, all 27 found a significant association, with none of them finding evidence for decreased aggression. Associations with corporal punishment were also found to be related to a number of *adult* outcomes including adult aggression, criminal behavior, and child abuse perpetrated by that person on their own children. Furthermore, when they looked at the studies that separated spanking from harsher forms of physical punishment, there remained a significant association between spanking and negative child behavior, albeit at less magnitude than the association found with more severe parental behavior. They also found that the links between spanking and worse child behavior were not significantly different in more methodologically rigorous longitudinal studies in comparison to cross-sectional ones that looked at only one moment in time. This is important because these longitudinal studies are better equipped to disentangle the effect of more defiant children *eliciting* more spanking from the effect of spanking leading to more defiant behavior (recall this was a criticism that was legitimately leveled against many of the cross-sectional studies).[24]

Did this study satisfy the critics and put the issue of spanking once and for all to rest? Of course not. The American College of Pediatricians continues to maintain that the research on spanking, including Gershoff's 2016 meta-analysis, remains severely flawed and misleading.[25] The critique cites four small studies, all at least 20 years old and all conducted by the same author, as evidence that spanking is effective when taught properly. These studies, however, focused on comparing spanking to other methods when a young child defied a time-out. And while spanking did improve child behavior in the short term, it generally was not found to be superior to a nonspanking condition, such as placing the child in their room.[26] As the authors from one of these studies states in their summary, "physical punishment did not appear to be a critical component" of their overall approach.[27] In the end, if these studies supposedly constitute the strongest scientific evidence *for* spanking, proponents of corporal punishment looking for research backing have their work cut out for them.

This is not to say that their criticism of the current spanking data is completely off the mark. Since more disobedient and oppositional kids tend to force parents to intervene more frequently, nonexperimental studies will tend to show that increased use of *any* kind of specific disciplinary technique is associated with more negative child behavior rather than less[28] because (i) the little angels who are temperamentally less aggressive and defiant by nature don't push parents to need to punish them very often, and (ii) all of our disciplinary strategies tend to yield temporary and imperfect results so it is unlikely that we see a pattern in which a parent uses a particular method once or twice and then gets to sit back and coast after that.

## Summary of the Spanking Literature

Putting all of these studies together, it is fair to say that the research evidence to suggest that spanking children leads to a variety of negative outcomes is large, mostly consistent, and imperfect. These negative outcomes cover a lot of territory and include higher levels of aggression, lower self-esteem, more strained parent–child relationships, less internalization of morality, and more mental health problems in the future. A recent study also linked early spanking to later dating violence.[29] And while much of this literature suffers from some methodological flaws that impede the ability to make a definitive conclusion regarding especially the effects of infrequent and calmly applied spanking, what may be even more remarkable about the spanking research is the nearly complete absence of any research that demonstrates it does anything *positive*. Overall, those that want to claim that spanking is a good thing to do with children need to look to somewhere other than the scientific data to support that claim, as the research literature as a whole suggests that corporal punishment tends to make the things that parents are using it for worse, not better.[30] Sure, it is possible to find very well-adjusted kids who were spanked, but it is just as possible that those children never needed that level of punishment in the first place.

As for the claim that society's softer approach to discipline has resulted in a generation of unruly youth with no respect for others, there is actually little indication of this. Rather, there are multiple lines of research to suggest that our newest generation of youth get into trouble *less* with their parents and the law than their predecessors. The number of kids in juvenile rehabilitation centers (formerly known as juvenile detention centers) is at the lowest levels in decades. Furthermore, there is increasing evidence that things like bullying, peer-to-peer assaults, and other types of disruptive and disobedient behavior are actually falling, despite some horrible events that capture both our hearts and our headlines.[31] Indeed, the dip in these kinds of behaviors has been interpreted by some as a *bad* thing, reflective of a new generation who have opted out of their age-appropriate rebellions of authority to hang out at home with their smartphones.[32]

Alex's pediatrician, who is well informed about the research on child discipline, cautions Melissa and Bill about using corporeal punishment as a way to reduce aggression and tells them that the research suggests spanking will likely only make things worse. She refers the family to a child psychologist who implements an evidence-based parent training program, which includes a number of elements including praising positive behavior, ignoring lower-level misbehavior, and occasional use of time-outs. Alex's behavior improves, although he remains more challenging than his brother, and Melissa in particular is grateful that they were able to avoid corporeal punishment.

## It Depends Factors

In many ways, the "It Depends" section for this chapter feels different than it does for some others and perhaps needs to be reframed from looking at variables that might be related to spanking being beneficial to variables that might be related to spanking being *particularly* harmful. With that qualification in mind, however, here are some factors that have been shown to modify the impact of corporal punishment on child behavior.

## Child Age

One of those factors certainly seems to be age, with even the more "pro-spanking" advocates noting that the practice should begin to get phased out by around age 6 and "rarely, if ever" used for kids older than 10 years old.[33]

## Spanking Frequency and Intensity

Another important factor relates to the frequency and severity of spanking, with the idea that there is a real difference between spanking that occurs on the bottom once a year versus frequent strikes on different parts of the body that occur on a more regular basis. Indeed, this distinction, which has been poorly made in some of the research studies on corporal punishment, has been a crux of the criticism against much of the scientific literature on the subject. In the first Gershoff review,[17] only 5% of the studies actually measured both the frequency and the severity of corporal punishment, with some studies simply categorizing families that never spanked and families that did, regardless of whether that meant once a year or once a day. As previously mentioned, future reviews tried to focus in on the importance of spanking frequency and, when they did, found evidence that when it occurred more regularly and as the go-to method of punishment, there were stronger associations with negative behaviors later in life.

## Child Perceptions of Corporal Punishment

Children can have very different views regarding the degree to which they see spanking as "normal" parenting behavior that is done for their own good. As a result, one could well imagine that the interpretation of being spanked as something that all loving parents do to keep their children on track might have a different impact relative to the interpretation that spanking is the action of mean and atypical adults who are acting outside of the mainstream. These different perceptions, in turn, could be related to cultural factors and the degree to which spanking is or is not accepted as a legitimate part of child-rearing.

Investigating this question can get a little tricky politically, and most studies have chosen to ignore the issue altogether. Some haven't, however, and those that do venture into this territory have found some interesting, although not entirely consistent, results.[30] While certainly there are ethnic and cultural differences regarding the rate of spanking and the degree to which it is accepted as standard practice,[34] there are mixed results regarding the question as to whether the established link between corporal punishment and negative child outcomes holds for all cultural groups. Some studies, for example, find less negative impacts of spanking in African American families compared to white ones,[35-38] with one study even showing that spanking early in life was related to lower levels of problem behavior in adolescence.[38] Other investigations, however, find that the association holds regardless of ethnicity.[39-41]

In trying to explain this inconsistency, one hypothesis is that the decisive factors are less about culture per se and more about other dimensions such as parental warmth or whether or not children feel accepted by parents who spank them. One study of older children (aged 9–16) was conducted on the island of St. Kitts, where corporal punishment, at least at the time, was generally viewed as "good, appropriate, and responsible parenting."[42] Like many other studies, they found a strong association between the amount of corporal punishment and child maladjustment. This link was diminished, however, among kids who didn't feel rejected by their parents in the process. Subsequent studies in other groups by some of the same researchers found similar results, namely that it was a child's sense of being accepted rather than rejected by his parents that was the important factor in the degree to which corporal punishment was associated with negative outcomes.[43]

Along similar lines, a longitudinal study conducted when groups of European-American, Africa-American, and Hispanic children were 4- to 5-years-old showed that, for all ethnic groups, spanking was related to later child behavior problems. However, the link no longer was present after statistically taking into account the level of emotional support the mother gave to her children.[39] Another recent study found a similar result.[44] Taken together, these studies suggest that there can be cultural differences in the link between corporal punishment and negative behavior, which, in turn, may be related to the amount of warmth and emotional support that children feel from parents who also use spanking. With few exceptions, however, it is important to note that these other factors didn't *negate or reverse* the associations between corporal punishment and negative child behaviors; it just made them not as strong.

## Child Temperament

There are at least a couple ways that child temperament dimensions can also be complicating this picture. One is that kids who are born with temperamental dispositions to have more negative emotionality and aggression are more likely to remain this way later in life. Studies have shown that these traits can be measured in infancy and that they remain somewhat stable as children enter preschool age.[37] Since these kids are also the ones who are more likely to receive harsher disciplinary behavior because of those traits, especially among parents who share their child's temperamental proclivities, what is actually a genetic effect (genes in the parents for negative emotionality and aggressiveness being passed to the child) looks like an effect of the parenting behavior itself.[45] In more technical terms, this is known as a passive genetic–environmental correlation.[46]

> Carla's parents do get another opinion for how to help their daughter, and this clinician is able to take a broader look at Carla's behavior and the many causes behind her anxiety and disruptive behavior. He explains to the parents that the spanking is unlikely to be the primary cause of Carla's anxiety but is probably not particularly helpful either. Together, they build some strategies designed to lower Carla's level of anxiety, which might be driving some of her angry outbursts. They agree to suspend the use of spanking for a while to see if things can get better with other disciplinary techniques. Three months later, Carla feels less anxious and the parents no longer see misbehavior that in the past would have provoked a spanking.

Along the same lines, another hypothesis that has been brought up earlier is that the harsher discipline in the lives of these more irritable and defiant kids comes from the children *precipitating* these responses in the parents (this is called an evocative genetic–environmental correlation or, if you are a strong antispanking advocate, blaming the victim).[47] Both of these scenarios can produce the illusion that it is the corporeal punishment itself that is the important causal factor in the child's worsening behavior when really other factors like genes are the primary culprit. These meddling complexities have certainly been noticed and described by some of the critics who believe that the negative effects of spanking have been overblown,[24] and they likely do play a role in making some of the spanking studies look more dramatic than they are. On the other hand, some of the more methodologically rigorous studies have tried to account for these complicating issues. It also is worth noting that if corporeal punishment was really that awesome in improving child behavior, we wouldn't need to be trying to disentangle all of these competing hypotheses for why spanking keeps getting associated with worse child behavior in the first place.

It is also possible that the corporal punishment itself has a stronger negative impact on kids with particular temperamental traits. Unfortunately, most studies haven't looked at this possibility, preferring to treat early child behavior as a factor to *control for* statistically rather than testing temperament as a factor that might prove to *change the effect* of spanking for some children. For example, we might envision a scenario in which kids who temperamentally tend to be aggressive become even more so when spanked in kind of a viscous cycle that gets perpetuated over time. Indeed, it seems highly likely that this is what most of the long-term studies on spanking are actually suggesting since these are the kids usually getting spanked the most. A study of 9-year-old Chinese children found that while harsher parenting was overall related to higher levels of child aggression, this was most prominent among children who temperamentally were high in the trait of sensation-seeking.[48] We could also imagine that more fearful children like those in the anxious category might easily become overwhelmed when spanked. Indeed, one study did show that spanking was related to higher levels of child aggression particularly among those kids who were rated higher in the trait of fearfulness.[49]

## It Depends Conclusions

Several "it depends" factors reviewed here converge to illustrate that some of them may render corporal punishment as particularly problematic or somewhat less so, with none actually tilting the scales to move in the opposite direction. Corporal punishment that is used infrequently and only with younger children shows weaker links with later child behavioral problems than when it is used regularly and with older kids. There also seems to be a protective effect among families who spank if the child also has a lot of positive interactions with the family and feels accepted by the parents. Finally, kids who tend to be more angry and anxious temperamentally appear to be especially prone to having those traits amplified in the context of corporal punishment. These factors are important things to keep in mind if you are determined to continue to keep spanking as an option in your family despite all this research or if you are not in a position to change a family's stance on this issue. Overall, however, it seems quite clear, even with all the "it depends" factors in play, that there remains a dearth of scientific evidence that corporeal punishment leads to anything good for a child over the long haul.

It also is worth pointing out that the research problem of trying to draw the line between "appropriate" spanking and abuse can play out with individual families as well. Yes, there are many parents who do spank and who are able to follow very clear parameters for when and how they do it, but the research tells us that there are also those who can be prone to using it too often and too aggressively when fuses are short and emotions are running hot. If in taking a hard and honest look at your own temperament as a parent you find yourself acknowledging that you may be one of those people who can lose their cool and wind up treating your children in ways you later regret, there may be some advantages to you forming a blanket "no spanking" policy in your household that is simple and probably easier to follow than a more flexible approach that requires you to think through a lot of options during times that clear thinking may be hard to access. As described in chapter 3, this may well be one of those times where it makes a lot of sense to move your parenting approach *away* from what feels most natural to you.

## Are Time-Outs Toxic?

As more and more parents take stock of the research conclusions and move spanking off the list of available options, a logical question that comes next is *what exactly should take its place*? For many, that alternative has been the time-out, in which a child who has committed a more serious offense is sent to a chair in a boring part of the house to sit alone for a matter of minutes before rejoining the family. This technique has now been incorporated into a number of evidence-based behavioral programs for children who struggle with aggression and rule-breaking with good results.[50,51] Lately, however, this supposedly kinder and gentler alternative to spanking has come under fire itself for being too harsh. Opponents decry time-outs as a form of parental neglect that abandons children at times of great need. Popular author and child psychiatrist Daniel Siegel wrote "Time-Outs Are Hurting Your Child" in a *Time Magazine* article[52] while promoting his *No Drama Discipline* book.[53] In trying to provide evidence for his position, however, he unfortunately used the same trick some of the anti–sleep training folks like to use by referencing neuroscience data on the effects of trauma that had nothing to do with time-outs specifically (unless you already equate time-outs with trauma). In response to some public criticism about the article, he later walked back these claims a bit in his blog in saying that what he meant was that he is opposed to "inappropriate" use of time-outs.[54]

What Siegel and many others argue is that children should instead be subjected to "time-ins" when they misbehave in which a parent moves closer to the child, listens to what is upsetting him, reflects those feelings back, and coaches the child back into a state of equilibrium. This approach has resonated with a lot of parents, some of whom with temperaments that are in many ways opposite to those who find spanking to be quite appealing. For these mothers and fathers (and I'd consider myself to be in this category), enforcing any kind of discrete punishment is tough, and endorsements to do away with them altogether are heartily welcomed and accepted. Unfortunately, however, research on the effectiveness of punishment-free parenting, especially for more behaviorally challenging kids, hasn't moved well past the "it worked for my kids" anecdotes[55] and personal opinions of some child experts. Studies that do exist are bogged down in some of the same methodological flaws as the spanking research, particularly the phenomenon that children who tend not to misbehave evoke less of *any* kind of systematic disciplinary measures. Of course, the no-drama advocates might point to this finding as evidence that all punishment methods don't do anything other than make parents feels like they've done *something* to address their child's behavior, and we'd be better off without the whole lot of them.

So what should a well-meaning scientifically-informed parent do? Not surprisingly, the answer might be to apply some good "one size does not fit all thinking" to the mixed messages we receive. To illustrate this point, consider the following two examples.

> Four-year-old Mikaela is known to "push people's buttons," and her single mother, Kelly, is having none of it. Unfortunately, her very frequent attempts to discipline Mikaela when she breaks the rules often don't seem to work. In an effort to avoid spanking, Kelly uses time-outs, *a lot*. The procedure usually involves Kelly telling Makaela that she is now in time-out for 4 minutes (1 minute per age) at which time Makaela will often simply refuse or take an extremely circuitous route to the time-out chair. She also usually defies the instruction to be quiet by singing as loudly as possible. If Mikaela gets out of her chair early, Kelly has been instructed to put her back in it, which she sometimes has to do several times. This has occasionally resulted in physical scuffles that make everyone more upset. Kelly wonders if there might be another way.

And now this.

> Andre is a 3-year-old boy who has been living with his foster mother for about 18 months. Sadly, Andre had to be removed from his birth parents' home due to substantiated charges of physical abuse and neglect. The foster mother has worked very hard with Andre, who can get quite aggressive at times and is prone to major outbursts that are hard to control. The use of corporal punishment has been strongly discouraged due to Andre's past, so the foster mother uses time-outs instead. However, doing do often results in Andre becoming even more out of control. During a time-out, Andre will scream out for his foster mother and cry intensely. The foster mother tries to ignore him but feels guilty in doing so when she sees the level of distress that time-outs seem to cause.

These two examples illustrate the degree to which different forces can be at play both with regard to why children misbehave and how they respond to the same intervention. Some children really do like to "test the limits" and can be more deliberate in their defiance. For other kids, there is underlying anxiety and worries about abandonment that can get easily activated and lead to meltdowns that looks more intentional than they are. For these children, the withdrawal of attention and imposing of strict punishment "teaches" them little and often can make the behaviors worse over time. Recognizing the difference between these two children helps craft a more customized response.

Mikaela appears temperamentally to be more of the confident type, and time-outs are provoking her to engage in a power struggle with her mother. She certainly doesn't like the time-out, but does not find them frightening. As a result, a good next step here is not to end time-outs as an option but to help the mother use them more effectively. Kelly might benefit from recommendations to use time-outs less frequently and reserve them for higher-level offenses like hitting others. Then, when she does use them, she should tell Mikaela that if she does not follow the time-out rules, something under Kelly's full control will be taken away instead (like screen time). This backup plan is preferable to Kelly physically restraining her daughter to get her to comply in time-out. With time, Mikaela realizes that 4 minutes in time-out is a better option than losing her privileges and she begins to willingly, but still begrudgingly, sit quietly when they are infrequently used.

For Andre, however, things are different. He might be very well be considered to be in the agitated category temperamentally, a profile that is often associated with kids who have a lot of early trauma in their past. To him, time-outs are not annoying, they are terrifying. His brain and body respond as though he is about to be hurt or abandoned again, and he loses any ability to control his emotions. For Andre, time-outs are best left out of the toolbox for when he misbehaves, and his foster mother does better to engage with Andre and help him learn better coping skills when he begins to get upset.

Research is slowly beginning to provide some data about the need for "it depends" thinking in these kinds of situations. One study, for example, showed that parents who were more restrictive in their approach to a child's misbehavior, meaning that they were more apt to scold and warn, fared better in the long-run with regard to lower levels of child defiant behavior but only if the kids tended to be more oppositional from the start. If they weren't, the same more heavy-handed approach tended to make things worse.[56]

Overall, then, it seems fair to say that a categorical proclamation that time-outs are universally unnecessary and neurotoxic goes *far* beyond the known science. While supportive parental engagement may be very useful for a highly emotional child who often has trouble calming himself down,[57] for another child it can teach him that breaking the rules results in some really nice one-to-one time with mommy. Time-outs are probably not that effective and may be counterproductive if they are getting used multiple times a day, if physical struggles ensue from trying to get a child to stay in time-out, or if they are being used for relatively minor infractions. Instead, they should be imposed infrequently and for more significant transgressions such as physical aggression. If a child refuses to stay in his chair, then time can be added to the time-out or, if that doesn't work, a privilege can be taken away in its place. Wrestling matches to keep a child in time-out are best avoided. Further, if a child has "lost it" and has become completely dysregulated, this suggests the need for a parent to engage rather than disengage by helping him learn methods to soothe and calm himself. As described in the opening chapter, the big picture here is to move away from global policy statements on parenting and toward a more flexible and scientific approach to what is and what is not working in our own little experiment that we call our family.

## It Depends—Discipline

**General Summary**

The vast majority of scientific evidence indicates that spanking is ineffective and is related to a number of negative child outcomes including increased mental health problems, poorer parent–child relationships, and higher levels of aggression later in life.

| "It Depends" Factors | Adjustments |
| --- | --- |
| Age | Spanking children over the age of 6 is related to worse child outcomes |
| Emotional support and acceptance from parents | Higher levels may reduce the negative effects of spanking |
| Child temperament—anxious and agitated type | These children may be particularly susceptible to react negatively to harsher disciplinary methods such as corporeal punishment |

# 11

# iToddler

## The Effects of Early Media and Technology Use

Some of you may not remember what screen time meant for young children in the simpler era of yesteryear. First, that term *screen time* didn't even exist because there weren't different types of screens to distinguish; there was just one—that big box, sitting in the living room. Programming, meanwhile, consisted of *Sesame Street, Mister Rogers,* and, if you were lucky, the chance to watch Tom and Jerry attack and maim each other on Saturday mornings.

Ah, how things have changed. Movies and television shows became available to own first on videotapes, then DVDs, and now as downloads or streamed right to one's television, phone, or tablet. Cable and then satellite companies helped increase the number of available channels from 3 to over 300. Video games emerged from a simple game of "pong" to visually spectacular and immersive worlds with missions you can play online against people across the world. And all of it now fits into the palm of our hands to access whenever and wherever we want it.

Eternal bliss, right? Not exactly. In my clinical practice, I can tell you confidently that conflict over screen time is easily the number one battleground between parents and children of all ages. And it's no wonder that this is the case. Seeing a toddler zone out in front of an iPad on a beautiful sunny day or re-enact the swordfight he just saw on *Lego Star Wars* against his little sister is going to cause at least some trepidation for most parents. Many people are quite worried, viewing screen time as nearly apocalyptic for the current generation. A recent article in *The Atlantic* by psychologist Jean Twenge was entitled, "Have Smartphones Destroyed a Generation?"[1] And the answer was yes, using

Chapter illustrations drawn by Jaq Fagnant

*Parenting Made Complicated.* David C. Rettew, Oxford University Press (2021). © Oxford University Press.
DOI: 10.1093/oso/9780197550977.003.0011

some data to conclude that smartphones are putting youth "on the brink of the worst mental health crisis in decades."[1] A widely viewed *60 Minutes* segment in December 2018 also conveyed serious concerns about the ways that screens may be negatively altering brain development.[2]

Yet others see media use as either no big deal or even a new digital reality that parents should be encouraging our kids to master as soon as possible.[3] Do screens really make attentions spans worse, help some children read, or cause sweet toddlers to become irritable and aggressive? Does the amount of time or specific content of the media really matter? And what kinds of kids might be most susceptible to these effects? These questions and more will be addressed in this chapter on the behavioral and cognitive effects of early screen time. The overall hope is that if you are going to be forced to fight over this issue for the next 15 or so years, you might as well be armed with as much reliable information as possible.

## It's Not Too Early to Make a Strategy

Many parents of infants and young children are well aware of the debates related to media use but feel like this is one of those things to put on the back burner and worry about later. Sure smartphones are completely altering the human race, you might be thinking, but my toddler still can't stand to be without me for more than 10 seconds. How worried do you need to be about texting and driving, after all, when your preschooler can neither reach the car pedals nor spell?

Some of these media-related parenting dilemmas do indeed play out more intensely with older children and adolescents, but these issues certainly are relevant for children under 5. As we'll soon see, toddlers and preschoolers are active little consumers of many different types of media already, and habits learned early can gain momentum as children grow.

> Aaron is a 4-year-old boy with two older siblings. Since infancy, he's been quite drawn to screens whenever one is around. His parents often find Aaron snuggled up for long periods of time with his older brother or sister watching the same tablet or television. They try to engage Aaron in other activities, but he often just doesn't seem that interested. At times, it's like he doesn't even know what to do other than watch screens. At the last annual well-check, the pediatrician asked Aaron's mother how much screen time Aaron consumed and she had to admit that she wasn't really sure. She also was a bit taken aback when the pediatrician began talking about some health risks associated with excessive screen time and wondered if the doctor was being overly alarmist, as, in her view, Aaron's interest in screens appears to be in line with most of his peers.

**Table 11.1**  Screen Use Recommendations for Young Children[4]

| Age | Recommendation |
| --- | --- |
| 0 to 18 months | No screens other than for communication such as video calls |
| 18 to 24 months | May begin to introduce high-quality educational programming to be watched with parent |
| 24 to 60 months | Maximum 1 hour per day total and none during meals or right before bedtime |

## The Official Recommendations

In late 2016, The American Academy of Pediatrics (AAP) revised its long-standing recommendations regarding media use for children 5 years and younger.[4] The AAP tried to balance their recommendations between the ever-changing science of developing brains and the practical realities of the modern world. As shown in Table 11.1, they continued their recommendation of no screen time for children under 18 months of age (except for video calls to grandma, of course!), arguing that very young children are not yet capable of reaping the benefits from technology and instead need "hands-on exploration and social interaction" to develop their skills.

The group, however, removed the no screens before age 2 recommendation by stating that digital media could be introduced for young children between 18 to 24 months of age as long as parents were present during viewing and the content featured high-quality programming. From ages 2 to 5, the previous limit of 2 hours per day total was lowered to 1 hour per day, again for educationally valuable shows. These guidelines are outlined in Table 11.1.

The response to these guidelines over the past few years has ranged from a hearty welcome to wondering what planet the authors of these recommendations were from. Some applauded the relaxation of the screen ban for children under 2 given the changing landscape of more interactive media specifically developed for young children,[5] while other complained that the guidelines remained overly restrictive and unsupported by the scientific data.[6]

Andrea is 3 years old and temperamentally on the nervous side. She has an interest in screens but not overly so, as best her parents can tell. Her parents try to keep her screen time to no more than an hour per day with the exception of the occasional movie night. They also try to make sure that the content is appropriate for someone her age. Unfortunately, however, Andrea had some trouble after watching the movie *Frozen*, and now voices some worry at night when she goes to bed about monstrous snowmen attacking their home. The parents feel badly about accidently introducing this fear and wonder if they need to rethink their screen policy.

## How Much Do Kids Actually Watch?

According to a 2013 report from the group Common Sense Media, the total screen time of children between the ages of 2 and 4 is just under 2 hours per day (1 hour and 55 minutes) while children from zero to 1 spend just under 1 hour per day on average. These numbers actually represent a slight decrease of 21 minutes from 2011.[7] Time on mobile devices has increased but is countered by decreases in "traditional" media sources like television. A total of 38% of children under 2 have used a mobile device to view media. In comparison, this same survey found that 40% of respondents did *not* read to their child at least once per day.

A few other statistics are relevant here: nearly a quarter or parents report that they let their young child watch the shows that they are watching, while 7% state that their child under 8 is allowed to watch "adult" shows. Despite the AAP admonitions, 37% of children between the ages of 2 to 4 have a television in their bedroom, although this varies by household income level with the rate being 56% in the *lowest* income group and 21% in the highest. There are also some differences by race/ethnicity, independent of income status, with African American children watching more television and being more likely to live in a home in which the television is generally left on during the day.

## The Controversy

### Potential Risks of Screens

The intellectual war over kids and screen time has many fronts. Those sounding the alarm over the negative effects of excessive screen time and media use describe a number of specific concerns.

1. Increased child aggression and emotional desensitization to human suffering due to exposure to violent media and video games
2. Reduced cognitive abilities and attention spans or even attention-deficit/ hyperactivity disorder (ADHD; this concern also relates to the erosion of other generally desirable personality traits such grit and perseverance)

3. The idea that screens are basically a huge waste of time and takes kids away from engagement in much more meaningful and productive activities. Using a nutritional analogy, screens are the brain equivalent of empty calories.
4. Increased anxiety from watching frightening content
5. Negative impacts on self-esteem and body image
6. Exposure to manipulative advertising
7. Safety concerns due to things like distracted driving
8. The modeling and glorification of bad behavior and bad choices like smoking and misogynistic attitudes toward women

For this chapter, we'll focus mainly on the first four items, as these arguably have the most direct relevance to toddlers and preschoolers who are generally not texting, playing *Call of Duty*, or watching *Game of Thrones*. In some ways, the concerns can be boiled down to those regarding the *quantity* of screen time, regardless of what it is, and those regarding the effects of specific media *content* (like violence) on a child's development.

John is a very challenging 5-year-old boy who is prone to intense angry outbursts and mood swings that go from ecstatic to enraged in a matter of seconds. His single mother, who is also trying to raise an infant girl, finds that the considerable time John spends on his tablet can provide precious moments of peace and focus, even if there are sometimes huge battles over turning it off. John seems particularly drawn to shows that feature fighting and violence, and some older cousins have helped him download some more realistic video games he can play. John's mother isn't a fan of these games but wonders if they are helping him release some of that negative energy that might otherwise be targeted against her and her baby.

## The Nothingburger

While those taking the "pro-media" position are generally not demanding that 3-year-olds come in from playing outside so that they can do a session of *Fortnite* on their iPad, their views could be summed up along two lines of argument. The first might well be called "Chill out!" Ever since Elvis Presley jumped onstage to play rock 'n roll and gyrate his hips, there have been throngs of curmudgeons ready to declare that cultural changes are causing the next generation to go to hell in a handbasket, yet somehow, our society continues to produce lots of solid upstanding citizens. Just as watching *Popeye the Sailor Man* didn't create a generation of spinach-binging children, kids today are not going to become lifeless zombies or pillaging anarchists just because they see one on TV. The takeaway from this point of view is that you can always count on the present generation to lament and wax poetic about the mind corruption of the next cohort of children despite little evidence that the "good ole days" were really that much better.

The other case being put forth more in the last 25 years, as screens evolve from devices of leisure to indispensable tools for day-to-day functioning, is that technology is here to stay and kids can either get on board or be left behind. From this perspective, children getting up to speed quickly when it comes to things like computers and mobile technology is not something to be tolerated but rather actively promoted for their own good (and so your child can develop her own software by age 25, sell it to a multibillion Silicon Valley company at age 27, and then retire and buy you a big house in the Bahamas).

In addition to these more polarized viewpoints is, of course, the common view of the supposed "silent majority" that argues for some middle ground, namely that parents should allow and maybe even encourage their children to watch television, listen to popular music, play video games, and become proficient with technology in moderation with regard to both quantity and content. Like red wine (for adults), a little bit is probably not harmful, maybe even good for you, but once some threshold is passed, the negative effects begin to outweigh the positive ones.

## Let's Get to the Research

One major challenge in trying to decipher the research on screen time and media use relates to how it is counted. Studies that simply sum up total media time while ignoring content could easily water down any kind of more nuanced but still important associations. Classifying an hour of *Sesame Street* the same as an hour of a first-person shooter game hardly seems ideal. You could try separating educational from noneducational programming, but unfortunately the term *educational* is very much in the eye of the beholder. Like that vague but still strangely reassuring label of "natural" you might find on a food product, there are no universal or enforced qualifications. This means that the term gets applied both to content that has been well-researched as developmentally valuable and to that "educational" app that allows kids to *count* the number of zombies they have just killed.

Perhaps the biggest headache when it comes to understanding media research has to do with the classic chicken versus the egg problem. Sure, it seems quite plausible that attention spans could be shaped in young children by spending multiple hours per day on screens, but it is also quite possible that some kids have a personality that makes them particularly drawn to all the bells and whistles that media can offer in the first place. In this way, screen time is really a result of a more innate predisposition toward having attention problems or aggression, rather than a cause.

## Child Aggression and Violent Media

### The Catharsis Effect

One of the biggest areas of debate when it comes to media usage and kids relates to the possible association between screen violence and real violence. For years, an argument was made that exposure to violent media is actually good for kids because it reduces the impulse to act in this way when the show is over. This phenomenon was often called the *catharsis effect*. The logic behind this hypothesis is that children, like all human beings, naturally harbor a certain amount of aggressive urges. Like a boiling teapot, this energy builds up and needs to be released one way or another. By watching cartoons with a lot of violent acts or by playing a shoot-'em-up video game, these urges are discharged harmlessly rather than spilling out through real and more destructive channels.

Some of these ideas date back to people like Sigmund Freud and his theories, many of which have not withstood the test of time or scientific inquiry. Still, there is something reasonable sounding about this catharsis effect. Why couldn't aggression, just like hunger, be satiated? Indeed, one survey found that 45% of boys reported that they played video games to "get my anger out."[8] An opposing analogy for media effects on aggression, however, is something like fire, which gets *bigger* the more you feed it. This perspective would maintain that a child's level of arousal and anger rises when interacting with violent media and predicts that kids would be *more* likely to act aggressively after being involved with media, not less.

### Studies on Child Aggression and the Media

Research on the link between media and violence comes broadly in two types. The first are often clever and tightly controlled experiments where children are randomly selected into two groups with one briefly exposed to more violent stimuli and the other to nonviolent stimuli. The groups are then observed for a short period afterwards for levels of aggressive or antisocial behavior. While these studies could be considered to be more scientifically rigorous with respect to the methodology, people often question the applicability of these studies to real life. It's quite a leap, many would argue, to understand the Columbine shootings from the small increase in pushing and shoving that might be observed after children see an episode of *Power Rangers*. The other broad category of study does not experimentally manipulate media exposure but rather records what is happening naturalistically and looks for associations either at the same point in time or in the future. The researchers have parents fill out questionnaires about the amount and type of screen time and then look at associations between those variables and child behavioral problems such as fighting or talking back to teachers. These types of studies are better equipped to look at actual levels of more problematic behavior over longer periods of time but are easily critiqued as "flawed" for not being able offer true conclusions about causation due to things like the chicken and the egg problem noted earlier.

Some studies also try to dig a little deeper as to *why* the association between media violence and aggressive behavior might exist by testing a number of theories. One common explanation is that exposure to violent media results in increased aggressive impulses through a sort of anticatharsis effect, like the fire getting bigger analogy. Another way that violent media might impact a child's level of aggression is through a process called desensitization—a fancy way of saying that if you continually exposure yourself to something that initially upsets you, then you are likely to get less and less upset with subsequent exposures. Desensitization can be a great thing if you are anxious about something: indeed, it's an effective treatment for people with different types of phobias. However, desensitization can also make someone emotionally hardened to things that *should* provoke a more emotional response, such as seeing another person get hurt. A child who has become numb to seeing violence, the argument goes, will have less holding them back from acting violently themselves. Still another possible mechanism is modeling, which is to say that violent media demonstrates to kids that violence is an acceptable way to resolve conflict, especially if the person doing it on screen seems cool and popular.

One of the first and most influential studies on children imitating violence they see is often referred to as the Bobo Doll Experiment, which was conducted by psychologist Albert Bandura at Stanford University and published in 1961.[9] It actually didn't look at media influences but rather focused on how kids would behave after watching someone in person, in this case an otherwise pleasant research assistant, beat the crap out of an inflatable clown named Bobo. It turned out that those kids who watched this research assistant were much more likely to act violently toward poor Bobo themselves when given the opportunity. This classic study demonstrated the power of imitation and opened the door to similarly designed studies that involved exposure not to scientists behaving badly but to violence viewed on screens.

A much more recent version of the Bobo Doll study in 2017 involved about 100 kids between the ages of 8 and 12 who were shown various clips from PG-rated movies *The Rocketeer* and *National Treasure*, some of which were violent.[10] After watching the clips, the children were observed as they were given some free time in a room that contained both toys and a real but disabled .38 caliber handgun that was rigged to register each time the trigger was pulled. The children who watched the movie clips with gun violence had more violent play after the viewing. Perhaps most unsettling was that trigger pulls were 22 times more likely among kids who saw the gun violence on screen compared to those who didn't, including one child who pulled the trigger against the temple of another child in the study.

Many other studies have also found increases in levels of child aggression following exposure to violent media—so much so that there has now been research looking at the improvement of media habits as prevention or even treatment of aggressive behavior. One of the best examples of this was a study that actively tried to change the "media diet" in Seattle area families of 3- to 5 year-old children with the hopes of improving behavior.[11] Half of the families were randomized to receive an intervention that was designed to replace violent and noneducational television and videos with more developmentally healthy media through the use of home visits, follow-up phone calls, and suggestions of prosocial media for children to watch. The intervention produced the desired effect in modestly reducing exposure to violent media. Six months later, the children who had received the intervention had slightly but significantly lower problem behavior scores compared to the control group. The authors also found that the benefit was strongest among low-income boys.

An example of a naturalistic study was one that followed kids longitudinally from ages 4 through 11 and focused on bullying behavior.[12] The researchers found that at age 4, the future bullies watched 5.0 hours of television per day versus 3.2 hours for nonbullies. After taking into account other factors, like bullying behavior at age 4, their analysis showed that television viewing continued to show a small but statistically significant association to future bullying. A similarly designed study found a link not to being a bully but to being the victim of bullying.[13]

These kinds of studies, however, don't all find positive links between media watching or video game playing and aggression, especially when other important factors are taken into account.[14,15] Even studies that do show a link find that this association is certainly not present in everyone. After playing video games, many kids feel more angry, but others don't, and some may even feel less angry.[16] This inconsistency speaks to the fact that it is important to be your own little scientist for your own little kid.

It also speaks to the need to avoid putting too much stock in a single study and look at the whole research landscape. In 2015, the American Psychological Association published the results of a systematic review of video games done by their Task Force on Violent Media. Video games, especially violent ones, are less prominent in the lives of young children but still very much a part of the overall media diet.[7] Moreover, their more interactive nature compared to passively watching a television show or movie might cause video games to exert stronger effects developmentally. The task force reviewed 14 recent studies and found that 12 of them supported a link between violent video game usage and actual child aggression measured in different ways, from teacher reports of classroom behavior to experiments in which children had the opportunity to give hot sauce or noise blasts to each other. Associations were also found related to increases in negative thoughts, like inferring hostile intent in another person when there isn't any, and decreases in things like empathy and sensitivity. An important qualification, however, is that none of these studies involved young children. Overall, the group concluded that there was a "consistent relation between violent video game use and increases in aggressive behavior, aggressive cognitions, and aggressive affect and decreases in prosocial behavior, empathy, and sensitivity."[51] Another comprehensive review of hundreds of studies encompassing over 130,000 individuals concluded strongly that video games were a causal factor on actual aggressive thoughts, feelings, and behavior. It found evidence against the old catharsis effect for media, with a kid's body actually becoming more aroused into a fight-or-flight mode after viewing violence.[17] A reanalysis of these data found evidence that the strength of this association might have been inflated due to bias, although the link remained present.[18]

This back and forth over the *magnitude* of the effect of violent media has in some ways supplanted the older argument over whether exposure to violent media results in more or less actual aggression in children. While few now argue that watching Wile E. Coyote try to kill the Road Runner with various sorts of Acme merchandise will actually improve levels of child aggression, the "pro-media" position now tends to argue that the true causal effect of media is miniscule related to other more important factors such as genetics, parenting, and exposure to real-world trauma and adverse events.[14] Others, however, continue to maintain that media can be blamed for 10% of our society's violence[19] and that the link between violent media and aggressive behavior is on par with the risk between smoking and lung cancer.[20]

Putting this all together, it seems fair to say that exposure to violence in television shows and video games does not induce a catharsis effect for most kids, with the majority of scientific evidence actually showing the opposite effect. While not all studies find this result, there is enough converging data across many different kinds of studies (experimental, naturalistic, intervention) to conclude that overall there is a true link that is at least partially causal in nature. How strong this link is and to what degree this effect applies to all types of children, however, remain very much in question.

## Do Screens Cause ADHD?

It's hard to watch an otherwise lively toddler or preschooler become completely absorbed in a video to the exclusion of all other environmental stimuli and not get a little creeped out. The glazed look in his eyes and the blank expression on his face can easily make a parent think that something is wrong here, even if the video is providing some precious moments of peace and independence for the parent. Then there is often that period of irritability and reactivity that many kids display after stopping their screen time and coming out of, as the parent of one of my patients said, their "stupor." Yet most parents remember being raised on at least a modest diet of television and videos without the destruction of our brain's attentional system. We still (mostly) listened to our teachers at school and retained our ability to become engrossed in a good book.

So what does science actually know about the impact of television, video games, and the internet on a child's cognitive ability and attentional skills? The concern over the potential negative impact of media on a developing brain has been with us for a while, with many studies showing significant associations between increased screen time and an increased prevalence of symptoms related to ADHD.[21-24] The problem, of course, is that there are a number of other things besides a casual relation between screens and ADHD that could be accounting for this link, such as the previously mentioned possibility that the attention problems are there first and it is these kids who are particularly drawn to the stimulation that screens can provide.

Some studies, however, have been equipped to test various ways that screen time and attention problems may be related to each and still find evidence supporting a causal link.[25-27] In one of them, screen time beyond 3 hours per day was found to be associated with attention problems, but this study was particularly strong because the researchers assessed levels of attention problems *at an earlier time* and did not find that baseline levels of attention problems predicted more screen time, thereby addressing some of the chicken and egg dilemma. Broadening the scope beyond attention problems, a 2019 study examined the link between total screen time and early reading skills in 69 preschoolers who also underwent a brain scan.[28] The authors found a correlation between more screen time and lower language and reading scores, but this association lost statistical significance once household income was factored in. Looking at the children's brains, screen time was associated with lower levels of "microstructural integrity" in several brain areas that are known to be important for language and reading. This link, however, remained significant even after controlling for household income, leading the researchers to worry that aspects of screen use may lead to "suboptimal neurodevelopmental stimulation" in early childhood. Also related to academic skills, a study of young children from Quebec that examined television viewing at ages 2 and 4 found that levels of early screen time predicted not only poorer attention skills at age 7 but also things like lower math achievement and classroom engagement, even after controlling for early child and family characteristics.[13] More screens earlier in life also predicted a more sedentary lifestyle at age 7.

This last sentence brings up the important point that even a true link between excessive screen use and attention problems doesn't necessarily mean that watching *Teletubbies* has some direct neurotoxic effect on a child's brain (although my brain usually hurt watching this show). Instead, the problem may be more related to "displacement," which means that when kids are glued to their screens they are *not* doing other brain healthy activities such as getting exercise, interacting with parents, playing with friends, learning new skills, and the like. Supporting this idea was a 2018 study linking better global cognition at age 8 to 11 with being able to achieve the holy trifecta of good sleep (9–11 hours per day), adequate exercise (at least 60 minutes per day), and limited screen time (less than 2 hours per day), although screen time was also predictive of better cognitive function all by itself. In case you are suddenly feeling deficient as a parent, only 5% of the sample met all three benchmarks.[29]

Muddying the waters here are some emerging studies that suggest that at least certain types of computerized exercises might actually work as a *treatment* for people with attention problems, although these activities look a little different than what kids do with a typical video game.[30] Nonetheless, with more and more of today's world involving computers and much of modern training for everything from flying airplanes to driving a car now involving simulators that look suspiciously like video games, one easily wonders whether these things should be introduced early. The evidence so far, however, encourages us to wait and reassures us that kids will continue to be able to wow us with their racing and planetary protection skills even if these things are introduced a little later in development.

Another theory for *how* screen time translates into cognitive problems has to do with the raising of a child's arousal set point for paying attention.[22,31] In other words, after spending hours in front of bright lights and loud noises as brave heroes prevent marauding space aliens from destroying the planet, the stimulation level produced by a kindergarten teacher standing in front of a class and trying to get students to follow along in their math workbook just doesn't measure up. School, and other types of lower stimulation activities, start to feel really boring relative to exciting shows and video games, and a cycle begins in which that higher level of sensory input becomes required to keep the brain engaged. A recent study in which mice were given 6 hours a day of sensory overload came to a similar conclusion in trying to explain the changes the animals had both in terms of brain development and behavior.[32]

## Positive Effects of Media

Before launching into even more ways that media use and technology might be problematic for young children, it is probably worth spending some space on the evidence that some forms of media can have positive impacts on development. A number of studies have indicated that educational shows such as *Sesame Street* can improve literacy skills, some cognitive functions, and social behavior among 3- to 5-year-olds.[4] According to a well-publicized 2015 report from the National Bureau of Economic Research, the introduction of *Sesame Street* "generated a positive impact on educational outcomes through the early school years" that was on par with the positive effects of huge and much more expensive projects such as Head Start.[33] The cognitive and literacy gains apply to children across many countries and groups around the world but were found to be particularly strong among children from more disadvantaged backgrounds.[4,34] Yet despite the positive results, the report also documents a slowly declining audience that peaked around 1970 when it was estimated that about one-third of children watched the show (about the percentage of people in the country who view the Super Bowl each year).

As mentioned, even much maligned video games have been shown in some studies to improve things like special memory, processing speed, and some fine motor skills.[35,36] Some studies have shown that playing video games such as *Super Mario* grow areas in the brain such as the hippocampus and prefrontal cortex, which has generally been viewed as a good thing given their role in functions like planning, motor performance, and working memory.[37,38] Again, however, virtually none of this research has been conducted in very young children.

Unfortunately for some media companies, the evidence is less rosy for media such as the *Baby Einstein* video series and many other products that were targeted for children 2 years old and younger and were originally marketed as a tool to improve developmental skills.[39] An experimental trial of one of the videos, *Baby Wordsworth*, found no evidence that it improved language development[40] while another study showed that for every hour per day infants between the ages of 8 and 16 months of age watched these videos, there was a 17% drop on a vocabulary measure.[41] The Walt Disney Company, which bought *Baby Einstein* in 2001, actually issued refunds to parents in 2009 because of the misleading claims that plopping down an infant or toddler in front of a video will make them smarter. Rather, research has shown that whatever benefits are observed from media exposure in children this young come from parents interacting with their baby during the programming (so much for getting the laundry done).[42-44]

## Virtual Traumatization

I've always been a big *Star Wars* fan. As a 10-year-old boy, I went to see Episode IV in the theater and was absolutely mesmerized by the big moving yellow letters and the special effects of the starships in combat. When my oldest son was born, I wanted him to enjoy the saga as well and had a hard time waiting for him to be old enough to watch these PG and PG-13 movies. When he was about 3, I started to show him carefully selected scenes that I thought would not be too much for him. He loved them and asked for more, which I happily obliged. Then, more than 10 years later, he casually tells me how much he struggled with Darth Vader nightmares when he was younger. Thanks a lot child mental health expert Dad!

Luckily for my son (and my conscience), the nightmares stopped, and he is now a *Star Wars* fan himself. That aside, the story illustrates another way that media exposure can affect behavior—it can scare us. Research in this area has demonstrated that watching frightening images through the media, whether it be a made-up horror movie or news coverage of events such as the September 11 terrorist attacks, can produce anxiety and even some degree of posttraumatic symptoms.[45,46] These fear reactions can extend beyond the immediate period after viewing and, for some children, contribute to overall higher levels of anxiety and increased perceptions of the world as a dangerous and threatening place.[47]

## Starting Healthy Media Habits Early

Some parents reading this and becoming increasingly wary of what seems like impending battles over screen time might logically figure that limiting screens very early in life could make these struggles easier down the road. While it may take a little more personal investment initially to engage young children in nonscreen alternatives, perhaps there is a later pay-off in the form of a child and adolescent who is less drawn to media and more capable of regulating screens on her own. Better to set limits now when it is a little easier, the argument goes, so you don't have to physically pry a smartphone out of an adolescent's hands later.

Great plan, but do things really work that way? One study from Japan looked at television viewing trends from infancy to age 5 and found that the group with high television usage during infancy maintained its high utilization for several years while those with less initial exposure saw declines in use as they got older.[48] To the degree that infant screen time is a function of parental choice while 4- to 5-year-olds are *asking* to watch TV, this suggests that an early investment to limit screen time may make the battle a little less intense going forward. Another study that followed a group of young children from age 2 to 5 showed that the toddlers who used more screens ended up being more sedentary at age 5.[49] While the authors concluded that "reducing screen viewing time in early childhood might promote healthier behaviours and associated outcomes later in life,"[49p201] the study didn't actually demonstrate this, and we still need much more definitive proof that limiting screen time when kids are young helps them regulate their screen usage later on.

## It Depends Factors

So far, there seems to be fairly good scientific evidence to back up the recommendations made by the American Academy of Pediatrics and other groups to limit media exposure and screen time for young children. From increased aggressive behavior to high levels of anxiety to reduced attentional and other cognitive skills, the research on the whole supports the notion that these problems are causally associated with media exposure that is "too much" with regard to both time and content. This statement does not mean that screens are the primary culprit for every problem we see in youth today, but there is enough of various different types of evidence to conclude that as parents we can't simply shrug it off as unimportant.

At the same time, the research shows us how many moving parts there are in this equation and how perilous it can be to make broad-based conclusions in this debate. Many of those variables have to do with the media itself. Even within a particular genre like television shows, for example, there seems to be very real differences between the effects of carefully made educational programming and the latest action-packed cartoon.

Thus, there are also a lot of "it depends" variables to consider when it comes to the individual child and family that have been identified in the research. In recognizing this complexity, the Center on Media and Mental Health (http://cmch.tv/) expressly states on their website their goal with regard to video games is "to identify what types of kids, playing what types of games, under what circumstances, are most likely to be at risk of harm—or most likely to benefit." Indeed, many experts have moved on from looking at average effects of media usage to how different types of media affect different types of people according to their own nature and motivations.[50] Some of those important factors most relevant to younger children are discussed next.

## Disadvantaged Backgrounds

Similar to the studies reviewed earlier suggesting that the effects of both positive and negative parenting are magnified with temperamentally more challenging children, there seems to be a similar effect when it comes to positive and negative media and children from more economically disadvantaged backgrounds. As previously described, research indicates that the beneficial effects of watching quality shows like *Sesame Street* tend to be less pronounced in the child who attends a state-of-the art preschool and is already surrounded by stimulating materials and engaging teachers compared to the child whose family does not have the resources to provide the same level of environmental enrichment. Looking from the other side, some studies focusing on the negative effects of media have also found stronger links among children from more disadvantaged upbringings.

## Gender Differences

On average, boys tend to be more interested in screens than girls. When it comes to gender differences in susceptibility to the negative effects of media, however, the data don't tend to show particularly strong differentiations. The link between screen time and ADHD-type problems was found to be somewhat stronger for boys[25] while a review of the link between violent video games and aggression found that the association held for both boys and girls.[51] Overall, the sex or gender differences that have been found don't generally rise to the level of being a major "it depends" factor.

## Child Temperament

### Aggression
There are a number of indications that the effects of media, good and bad, might vary based on a child's temperament. Children differ temperamentally, for example, on their tendency to become angry and aggressive, and this trait has been found to be influenced to a significant degree by genetics.[52,53] Using the categories described in chapter 2, many of these children might be described as being of

the agitated type. A recent study, albeit in adults, compared behavior, physiology (blood pressure and pulse changes), and brain activity in relation to viewing violent media between a group of young men who had a history of aggression versus a group that didn't.[54] The authors found that the more aggressive group showed different reactions to the media in all three domains; for example, the blood pressure among those in the aggressive group went down with the viewing of violent media while in the other group it went up. This study is in line with research on personality traits suggesting that individuals who at baseline are higher in neuroticism (easily become anxious and angry) and lower in the trait of agreeableness (less cooperative and compassionate) and conscientiousness (less organized and goal-oriented) tend to be the most vulnerable to the effects of violent video games.[55] While not uniformly found in pediatric samples,[56] several studies have shown that increases in aggressive thoughts and behavior after playing video games or watching violent media are strongest among those children who are more aggressive and angry *before* the media exposure.[16,57] All this suggests that violent media has the potential to make things worse for kids who already tend to be more aggressive and hostile in the first place.

> For John, who likely fits into the agitated type with regard to his personality profile, it's unlikely that his high level of interest in more violent media is discharging his aggressive feelings as his mother was hoping. In fact, it could be making things worse as he becomes increasingly desensitized to violence while not engaging in other activities that could help him self-regulate better such as being physically active and having pro-social interactions with peers. Yet as John's mother increasingly realizes that screens are part of the problem rather than part of the solution, she grows nervous at the idea of having to impose limits that she knows won't come without a fight.

Anxious Kids

Like more aggressive children, kids who tend to be anxious can also see these traits expand due to their media habits. A study of Dutch 4-year-old children who were shown scary clips from the movie *Dinosaur* found that the strongest fear reactions, as measured by stress reactions on the skin similar to lie detector tests, were among children who had the combination of being both temperamentally fearful overall and who were found to be less securely attached to their mother.[58] For many children with the anxious personality type, then, the biggest problem from screens may not be increased aggression or decreased attention spans but rather the fueling of anxiety and the spreading of the belief that the world is a very dangerous place. For parents of these types of children, the concern may be less about the imitation of violence seen in a cartoon and more about not getting that kid into a bath for a month after glimpsing a choice scene from the movie *Jaws*.

Andrea's parents decide to focus on the scarier content of what Andrea is watching rather than the total amount of screen time. They spend more time thinking about what shows may be anxiety-provoking and shift toward more educational programming. When there is the possibility of a show generating some fear in Andrea, one of the parents now tries to be there with her to help put things in context (or change what they are watching).

The Little Home Body

There's another category of children who can also get easily sucked into excessive media use: a group that hasn't had as much airtime when it comes to some of the other topics covered in this book. These are the kids in the mellow personality cluster, who may not be particularly aggressive or particularly anxious but can lack a certain amount of motivation or industry to get involved in things. For these children, screens can feel like a wonderful activity because it doesn't require doing much—you sit there, get entertained, and maybe even enjoy a nice snack. In moderation, this probably doesn't cause too many problems, but unchecked these are the ones who can be content to do *a lot* of screen time at the expense of other activities that would be healthier to pursue. Over time, some of these children can find themselves at a complete loss of what to do with themselves other than look at screens.

## Ah, But Here's the Challenge

In reading these examples and hearing about the research on screens, a theme begins to emerge that reveals a major challenge for parents trying to keep their kid's screen time within reason: media habits don't *create* particular traits; they *reinforce* them. The children who are more inattentive by nature get easily pulled into all sensory bombardment of action videos and games and then, in turn, increasingly struggle to focus during more mundane activities. The children who are more prone to act aggressively really enjoy more violent media, which then pushes those predispositions further. Kids are not blank slates; they come into this world with momentum to behave in certain ways and often are masters at getting the environment to strengthen those tendencies. Kids who don't like to read, *don't* read, and then their skills lag further behind. Breaking these cycles can therefore be very difficult, especially when we consider the fact that we are asking these things of parents who may have exactly the same genetically influenced predispositions themselves. It's hard enough to parent an aggressive, impulsive child, and even more so if you tend to be an aggressive, impulsive parent. As Jim Hudziak, Director of Child Psychiatry at the University of Vermont Medical Center, often says, parenting decisions that have to be made with more temperamentally challenging children are "twice as hard, and twice as important."

## A Few Practical Suggestions

In recognition then that moderating a young child's screen time is a worthwhile but challenging endeavor because it often runs against their temperamental tide, it is probably worth saying more than, "Good luck with that!" Remember, the good news here is that you are starting early with these limits so your child will be much more likely to accept them as part of life. There still may be a hump to get over initially with these new rules, but that's much better than the mountain that is created by waiting until your child is a teenager. To get things started, here are some practical tips, as shown in Box 11.1.

> *"Go outside," is probably not enough.* To change behavior away from a reliance on screens, parental engagement is likely necessary. Keeping in mind that some kids really haven't learned how to keep themselves busy without screens, parents may need to help come up with alternatives and then do some of those things with them, at least at first. Siblings can also help here, especially if "no screen" time is synchronized for everyone at the same time.
> *Fight fire with fire.* By this I mean use a device's own technology to help you set reasonable limits on screen time and content. There are also products that can be deployed at the level of a Wi-Fi router to manage multiple devices. They do cost money and can take a little while to learn, but this investment

---

### Box 11.1  Tips to Help Regulate Your Child's Screen Time

- Participate with them in doing non-screen activities
- Make use of technologies that helps you limit screen time and content
- Have your child earn screen time by doing less preferred but healthy activities
- Watch at least some of the content with them
- Show some flexibility with more educationally valuable media
- View media use like any other acquired skill and actively teach it
- Model good screen use yourself

can be well worth it—especially when you get to have a *machine* telling your child their screen time is up rather than you (for the fourth time).

*Earn it.* The amazing pull of screens can be turned to an advantage when used as a motivator. If your child often resists playing outside, for example, maybe 30 minutes of active outside play earns her viewing of a 30-minute show. You can set the exact ratios in a way that works best. One caveat, however, is that this technique is probably best for activities that your child really does not have a natural interest in already. The reason is that the introduction of an external motivator like screens might take away some intrinsic motivation the child already has for the activity. If your child already likes to read, for example, having a child earn screen time by reading could make reading feel less inherently appealing. See chapter 8 on picky eating for more details about this phenomenon.

*Watch with them.* Especially when media content is the issue, it is important for parents to have a good idea of exactly what is being viewed. When watching shows or playing games together, there are opportunities to interact and discuss what is on the screen. Sharing the experience also helps parents learn about their child's media preferences and tastes, so that you can make better conclusions about how media is or isn't affecting *your* child. I know, I know—you may initially lose that golden time to get things done on your own, but don't worry, your child will likely want to see the *exact same thing* 100 more times if you need to catch up on those emails.

*Allow some extra flexibility for more educational content.* Remembering that not all screen time is equal, one suggestion for kids who are begging for some extra tablet time is to say yes but insist that the programming be educationally valuable as a way to interest your child in shows like *Sesame Street* or more skill-building content. When our then 6-year-old began to rebel against some fairly stringent screen time limits, we downloaded an app that showed him how to play chess and told him time on this app, within reason, wouldn't "count" toward his limits. While he's likely not the next Bobby Fisher, he learned to play the game and still enjoys it.

*Teach it.* We don't expect kids to just learn how to play baseball by themselves so why should we just leave kids alone to acquire media habits that will likely become a huge part of their modern life. Do some research on what shows to watch, what games and apps to use, and then *show* your child the ways that media use can enrich someone's life without it taking over.

*Don't Be a Hypocrite.* Even a 4-year-old can legitimately call you out for not practicing what you preach. Getting your child to look at an actual book is going to be much easier if she sees you looking at them, talking about them, and enjoying them too. Keep your own media use in check, especially when you are interacting with your child. The Facebook post will still be there, trust me.

## Summing Up

As we leave this vast area of research and opinion, there appears to be good cause to keep a young child's exposure to screens modest with regard to both time and content, even with the acknowledgment that screens are not the root of all evil in youth and will inevitably be a part of their world as they grow up. Increased aggression, anxiety, and attention problems all can be exacerbated with excessive and inappropriate screen exposure, and children who already may be heading in these directions are often the same ones who are particularly drawn to screens in the first place, thereby reinforcing these traits. At the same time, there is a fair level of inconsistency in the research that likely reflects that fact that there are a multitude of different reactions to different types of media, and which response your individual kid will have can't be predicted all that accurately from an average of 1000 4-year-olds in Australia (no offense to Australia). This doesn't mean that the research is worthless but does suggest that a parent may do best by starting with a reasonable media strategy that is informed by the science, observe what actually happens with an open mind, and be willing to modify that plan by the information coming back. If every request to your daughter to turn off the iPad results in a complete meltdown or if your son's viewing of *Spider Man* results in his younger sister nearly suffocating from being wrapped in cobwebs (i.e., blankets), it is time to rethink and retool. Conversely, if your preschooler seems to benefit from a reasonable video break after school before moving on to other activities, there's little to suggest that her viewing of some Pokémon battles will turn her into a serial killer. Simple, right? Learn—apply—observe—adjust. As straightforward as it sounds, getting the right media policy down for your kid is likely to be a source of trial and error for years to come. It is worth trying to get right, however, and starting early will give you the best chance of helping your children make the best use of media technology, and not the other way around.

## It Depends—Screen Use

### General Summary

A child's use and exposure to media affects brain development. These changes can be both positive and negative. While the magnitude of the effects remain a matter of debate, the majority of scientific evidence supports the view that excessive screen time and exposure to violent and developmentally inappropriate content can lead to increased child aggression, attention problems, anxiety, and other negative outcomes.

| "It Depends" Factors | Adjustments |
| --- | --- |
| Socioeconomically disadvantaged backgrounds | There is evidence that both the positive benefits from things like educational programming and the negative effects of media are more pronounced in children from disadvantaged backgrounds. |
| Aggressive children/agitated type | These children may be particularly susceptible to showing more aggression themselves with exposure to violent shows and video games. |
| Anxious type | These children may be particularly susceptible to becoming more anxious with exposure to violent media content. |
| Mellow type | These children might be particularly prone to excessive screen time at the exclusion of other activities. Parents may need to be active to help them find other activities to occupy their time. |

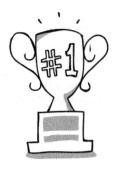

# 12

# Good Job!

## Science Examines Praising and Overpraising

Children from generations past were not coddled. Whether it be due to fears of spoiling children or simply from existing in a time in which parenting was considered less of a specific profession, one just didn't hear the frequency of "Good jobs!" and "Great work!" that now echo through many households and schools today. The change occurred several decades ago as the self-esteem movement gained popularity in the 1970s. In its wake came related cultural shifts such as efforts to downplay competition in sports and academics. But lately, as parents listen to the steady flow of compliments bestowed upon kids and watch all the players in Little League receive trophies just for showing up, there has been increasing concern that all this unbridled approval may be backfiring developmentally, particularly if it hasn't been truly earned. The original enthusiasm for the idea that praise builds strength and confidence has now been tempered with the worry that it can lead to too much focus on oneself, a lack of motivation to try harder, and, ironically, a sense of self that is *more* fragile and easily disrupted with even a minor critical comment. Some adults, I venture, also just find the continuous stream of praise to be incredibly annoying.

Has the self-esteem movement gone too far? Has our intention to help children feel valued and special created a praise junkie generation that quits at the first sign of trouble? While there is seemingly no end of opinions on this topic, actual data have slowly been accumulating. What the studies are now suggesting is that the issue is more complex, with plenty of "it depends" factors to consider regarding the individual child, parent, and even type of praise that is given.

Chapter illustrations drawn by Jaq Fagnant

*Parenting Made Complicated*. David C. Rettew, Oxford University Press (2021). © Oxford University Press.
DOI: 10.1093/oso/9780197550977.003.0012

Three-year-old Gabriella is cared for by her mother Juanita, who wants very much for her daughter to feel confident and valued as she grows up. Part of the strategy to accomplish this involves Juanita actively trying to give Gabriella compliments when she shows positive behavior. One day, when Gabriella's grandparents were visiting and hearing Juanita tell Gabriella that she was "so smart" and "so pretty," the grandfather spoke up against all the praise that Gabriella was receiving. "You know," he said to Juanita, "you are going to give her a big head with all those compliments, and then no one will want to be around her when she gets older." Juanita isn't so sure, but now has some doubts about her practice around giving praise.

Kids care what their parents think of them. The older ones may deny it, but most of them too will warm when their achievements and efforts are recognized with a kind word or gesture. My own father was pretty thrifty when it came both to money and compliments. When praise did come after a good grade or a big hit at a baseball game, it meant a lot. Many years later, I have to admit that I still respond very positively when I hear approving comments from others. As someone who has run a training program for young physicians pursuing child psychiatry as a specialty, I've also seen first-hand the wide range of emotional and behavioral responses to giving both positive and negative feedback. For some of my trainees, it becomes quite evident early on that hearing compliments is quite important and that any kind of constructive criticism needs to be presented gently. For others, I continue to be astonished at how impervious they are to the appraisals of their supervisors.

Mary is an admitted helicopter parent. She believes firmly that parenting is an active process and that it is important for parents to praise children when they are acting well and point out firmly when they aren't. This approach seemed to work okay for Mary's daughter who is now in the second grade, but 4-year-old Max is struggling. He is easily frustrated and quick to give up. Recently, he has also made some self-disparaging comments about not being good at various things. These behaviors and statements are starting to trouble Mary, and she wonders if being even more effusive with her praise will help.

Of course, the argument over praise in young children is, to a large extent, about degree. There aren't too many child experts out there advocating that parents shrug their shoulders and stare stone-faced like Olympic ice dance judges after a child has poured out his heart and soul on a project. And despite the stereotypes of helicopter-style parents, there also are few who believe children should be praised for breathing. Obviously, there is a lot of space between those extremes, which is why the whole topic of praise is so widely debated today. Most parents have no problem saying nice things about their daughter's beautifully drawn picture that took an hour of painstaking effort, but the proper response is a little murkier when she scribbles something down for 30 seconds and then says excitedly, "Look what I drew!"

## Praise as Reinforcement

The case in favor of more effusive praise comes from two main lines of reasoning and investigation, as shown in Table 12.1.

The first relates to praise as a form of *positive reinforcement*, which in the world of learning theory means a response that tends to make certain behaviors more likely to occur again in the future. Putting aside all the warm fuzzy aspects of saying nice things to your child, the idea here is that praise *works* to increase the likelihood that whatever behavior you are praising will happen again. When you say to your 3-year-old boy, "I love the way you were able to get dressed all by yourself today!" the cold calculation behind the statement is that doing so will provide some additional motivation for him to do the same thing tomorrow and, if you're lucky, might even generalize further to something as miraculous as tying his own shoes. The more praise, the logic follows, the more positive behaviors, as long as you have a child that actually finds praise to be rewarding.

It's worth noting that praise does not have to come in the form of a verbal compliment uttered during a time that a child is specifically looking for such a response. Hugs, high-fives, and little squeezes on the shoulder count as well. There also can be unexpected praise, which some child development experts believe can be especially powerful. These are moments that are easy to miss. A father, for example, who is trying to encourage his 4-year-old daughter to play on her own

Table 12.1 The Pros and Cons of Praise.

|  | Arguments For | Arguments Against |
|---|---|---|
| Praise as Reinforcement | Children like praise and so will be more likely to do things they are praised for | Praise quickly loses its value when given abundantly |
|  |  | Praise can replace more intrinsic motivations for accomplishment |
| Praise as Self-Esteem Builder | Praise builds an inner sense of value and efficacy which is needed to succeed in challenging situations | Excessive praise can lead to selfishness and feelings of superiority |
|  |  | Unearned praise sets up kids to fail when things get tougher |

once in a while, might not want to risk disturbing the peace when he realizes she is actually doing so in another room, but that may actually be an important moment to tell her how well she is doing.

Most critics concerned about overpraising don't deny the benefits of a good occasional "atta boy." Indeed, it is this reinforcing property of praise that they maintain gets cheapened and devalued when children are praised too much. Like any other type of currency, they argue, praise can become next to worthless when it is overly abundant. Thus, the only way to ensure that praise retains its potency as a reinforcer is to keep it something special. This argument can be extended to other types of rewards when given too liberally such as giving all players in a league a prize rather than just the winning team. A hard-earned trophy for being on the championship team gets put prominently on the top of the bookcase, while the participation medal gets stuffed in a drawer. Eventually, the concern is that not only does praise lose its power to promote excellence but what reinforcing properties it does retain end up encouraging mediocrity.

The other often mentioned problem with the reinforcement properties of praise is that it sucks away any intrinsic motivation for a particular behavior. Continuing with the baseball theme, the concern is that if a child is successfully motivated to practice and excel because of the praise that is coming, then he won't be motivated by other things such as an inner drive to improve or a natural love for the game itself. This, then, sets up a precarious situation when the child next year is assigned a coach who doesn't praise so much, and he now lacks these other motivations to continue playing. Some writers have indeed talked about our current society creating a generation of praise "addicts" who are prone to quit and become discouraged when those "Great jobs!" start to fade. In one widely read article, author of several books on education and childcare Alphie Kohn writes, "The more we reward people for doing something, the more they tend to lose interest in whatever they had to do to get the reward."[1]

Of course, those of you following these arguments closely might be starting to notice how some of these critiques of praise can contradict each other. If frequent praise causes it to become worthless, for example, then how do we create this generation of praise junkies who shrivel up as soon as the praise is removed? Here is where some real scientific evidence could be very valuable.

## Praise and Self-Esteem

The second major goal for praise is to act as a builder of self-esteem: a key ingredient in the development of a person who is happy, confident, and willing to go forth in this big bad world toward the pursuit of one's goals. Self-esteem refers to a person's inner sense of worth.[2] While the term dates back to a famous psychologist in the 1800s named William James, the concept was revived in the 1970s with books such as *The Psychology of Self Esteem* by Nathaniel Branden.[3] Many scholars at the time began viewing low self-esteem as one of our society's central challenges, underlying problems from criminal behavior to economic underachievement.[4] These ideas developed—some might say twisted—into the notion that a child's self-worth needed to be cultivated and nurtured through the words and actions by parents rather than simply being a *product* of success and accomplishment. This theory become widely popular among many prominent mental health professionals of the time, and it represented a real departure from earlier approaches to make sure kids "knew their place" (which generally meant at the bottom). In 1986, for example, the state government of California funded a task force at a quarter of a million dollars per year to make recommendations that might help raise the state's collective level of self-esteem in an effort to combat problems such as teen pregnancy, drug abuse, and even low state revenue.[5]

Since the new millennium, however, the fervor to view self-esteem as *the* critical factor to raising happy and successful children has waned. A comprehensive, albeit skeptical, review of the self-esteem literature was published in 2003 and concluded that the case for self-esteem as an important causal factor for all things good was much overstated, although the authors did note evidence for links especially between self-esteem and both happiness and persistence.[5] The research, however, has continued to churn and often does find links between low self-esteem and things like aggression and other kinds of antisocial behaviors[6,7] as well as to depression and anxiety.[8-11] There are also data demonstrating associations between increased self-esteem and higher levels of well-being and overall functioning,[12] even in non-Western societies that put less emphasis on individual achievement.[13]

This ongoing attention to the importance of self-esteem has not been missed by parents who have been told that providing praise is an important way of showing children that they are cherished and important. Fully 85% of parents, according to a 1999 survey, believe that they need to praise their child's intelligence to convince their kids that they are smart.[14] The basic premise is that a child who hears frequent praise will begin to internalize it, which, in turn, will create a strong and secure foundation of confidence that can come in very handy when the child faces challenges.

But self-esteem is not without its hazards. Too much of it can lead to a sense of superiority and entitlement. Even when it doesn't, self-esteem without substantive *skills and abilities* that enable someone truly to succeed can be a very fragile flower. Eminent psychologist Martin Seligman, who is widely credited as the founder of the positive psychology momentum and is no curmudgeon when it comes to exalted concepts such as happiness and optimism, has written that self-esteem is more of a barometer for how well someone is doing overall rather than an independent entity worth pursuing for its own sake. Breaking self-esteem into "doing well" and "feeling good" components, he worries that an empty appeal to the feeling good side will have little positive effect compared to teaching children *how* to succeed and be resilient under stress.[15]

## The Evidence for Praise

With all of these very rational sounding ideas floating around about the positive and negative effects of praise, there clearly is a need for some actual data to refute or support some of these claims. While we will soon see that the science about praising children very quickly moves to "it depends" factors, such as the type of praise and the type of child receiving the praise, a few more general conclusions can be reviewed first.

It is fair to say, as far as the major professional organizations go in pediatrics, psychology, and psychiatry, that encouraging parents to be generous with their praise is pretty standard fare from these established parenting authorities. The Centers for Disease Control and Prevention advocates for the use of praise in its websites and parenting videos,[16] as do groups such as the American Academy of Pediatrics,[17] American Psychological Association, and American Academy of Child and Adolescent Psychiatry.[18] Some of this encouragement is getting more nuanced as we'll discuss soon, but the overall message has been that praising children is an important tool to help reinforce positive behavior and help build a child's feeling of worth.

Much of the evidence for these endorsements comes from the large volume of scientific literature on overall positive parenting and the authoritative parenting style (see chapter 3).[19] Praise, along with other things like setting good limits and supporting children when upset, is literally a priori built into the definition of positive parenting and the rating scales that attempt to measure it.[20] While this research is compelling, the grouping of praise with other elements can make it hard to tease out the specific contribution that praise makes to the overall equation. One group that reviewed 41 different studies on the relations between praise (considered independently of other parenting behaviors) and child compliance (i.e., getting kids to display behavior that parents want) found "mixed" results that were less definitive than expected.[21] Specifically, the authors found that individual studies were quite inconsistent on whether or not they found a significant association between praise and more compliant behavior. Some did, and some didn't, and the researchers speculated that one reason may be that the positive effects of praise may take time to be fully realized. This review did not look at things like self-esteem and long-term functioning.

Another source of support for the use of praise comes from research-based programs that have been developed to help children who struggle with more oppositional and defiant behavior. These methods are often referred to in professional circles as "parent behavioral training" programs. One program that we use in our clinic for "strong willed" 2- to 6-year-olds directly teaches praising or verbal rewards as one of the core skills.[22] The authors argue strongly that using praise for behavior a parent would like to see more of does not erode other motivations for that behavior. They state, "Rewards don't destroy self-motivation, they enhance it,"[22p95] and they take a more developmental perspective on the issue by suggesting that people in general often need external rewards to begin doing things before the intrinsic rewards of the behaviors start to take over. An analogy here might be a person trying to eat better and lose weight who is motivated at first by people noticing the change in appearance and then, over time, starts to enjoy the feeling of a healthier body later on. Praise is similarly an important component of many other research-backed approaches to more challenging child behavior including protocols such as parent–child interaction therapy[23] and The Incredible Years.[24]

This modest support for praise in general, however, certainly doesn't confirm the idea that parents should simply be heaping it on at all times. Thus, we turn now to a somewhat newer line of evidence that suggests that, when it comes to praising children, there are a number of important "it depends" factors to keep in mind.

## It Depends

### Not All Praise Is Considered Equal

Many parents have already heard the message that, when a child misbehaves, there is a big difference between criticizing their *behavior* and criticizing *them*, and we, as informed parents, all do our best these days to remember to say that a child's action was "inappropriate" rather than calling them a "bad boy" or a "bad girl." In a nutshell, this is the same distinction being endorsed when it comes to how best to express praise and encouragement.

Researchers who study praise often divide it into two main types, as shown in Box 12.1.

The first is often referred to as *person praise*, which focuses on an individual's traits. Telling a child that she is "smart," "a great baseball player," or "so pretty" is person praise, because it says something about who the child *is*. By contrast, *process praise* focuses on more specific behaviors that lead to a successful result, such as effort or other strategies that help a child accomplish a goal. (There are other praise statements that don't fit neatly into these two boxes as well as short utterances like "Awesome!" or "Yay!" that defy easy categorization but the focus of research has been on person versus process praise.)

> **Box 12.1 Types of Praise**
>
> ---
>
> Person Praise: This type focuses on an individual's traits
> - Example: "You are so pretty!"
> - Example: "You are the smartest kid in the whole class!"
>
> Process Praise: This type focuses on specific choices or methods that a child use towards achieving a goal
> - Have your child earn screen time by doing less preferred but healthy activities
> - Example: "I love the way you didn't give up when you had those tougher math problems."
> - Example: "You slowed down and really focused to make this colorful drawing."

These two main types of praise have been shown to play an important role in how a child understands success and failure in themselves and in others, according to Stanford psychologist Carol Dweck and her colleagues who have been studying this phenomenon for years.[25] Their work has revealed that some children seem to approach the world with what they call a *fixed mindset* in which they believe that a person's accomplishments and successes are generally determined by factors outside of their control—like how much natural intelligence or innate talent someone has. Other kids, however, come to the table with more of an incremental or *growth mindset*, which holds that things like intelligence or sports abilities are malleable and can be obtained through effort and practice. There is evidence that differences in mindset are present in children as young as preschool age and that these beliefs can affect a child's motivation to work hard, especially as things start to get difficult.[26,27] When faced with a challenging task, people with more of a fixed mindset are more prone to give up, as they are worried that struggling with something *reveals* that they actually are not as smart or talented as everyone thinks they are. Those with a growth mindset, however, are more likely to seek out challenges as opportunities to build their skills and abilities.

As you might imagine, there has been a lot of buzz these days in schools across the globe on how to promote a growth mindset in children. One area of focus in particular has been in the way that praise and encouragement are delivered by teachers and parents alike. Consider again the example of a 3-year-old girl who spends an hour making a picture and then is eager to show the drawing to her mother. In responding, the mother has a number of available options. She might say something like, "Wow, you are really a great artist!" She might even go further and comment that her daughter is "the best drawer in the class." Alternatively, the mother might focus not on the person but the process that produced the drawing by stating something like, "You really worked hard to get this picture to be just right" or "I see you tried some new things in this picture." While you may recall having said something similar to all three of these responses at different times to your own child, it is worth stepping back to understand how these different praise statements might have different impacts relative to fixed and growth mindsets. The first two statements are examples of person praise as they convey something about the daughter's level of intrinsic talent that has been demonstrated in the drawing and thus could be seen as promoting a fixed mindset. The second statement in particular goes even further by the mother's *ranking* of her daughter's ability relative to others. These kinds of ranking statements convey to a child that not only are you paying attention to her, you are also paying attention to where she places relative to her peers. The last statements, by contrast, would be growth mindset promoting examples of process praise in that they highlight the effort and methods that went into the drawing.

Studies have supported the hypothesis that there is indeed a link between the type of praise a children hears and their view of success and accomplishment, with those who hear more process praise tending to develop more of a growth mindset and those who hear more person praise having more of a fixed mindset.[28-30] They further have shown that different types of praise can have different effects on a child's motivation level, especially when it comes to hanging in there after being presented with more challenging material.[31] In one study of kindergarteners, those who had received process praise during a role-play interaction with an adult showed more positivity and persistence when faced afterwards with a more demanding task, compared to children who had received either person praise or criticism of their work.[32]

Psychologist Liz Gunderson examined this question in a more naturalistic setting by having researchers go to the homes of children when they were 14, 26, and 38 months of age under the auspices of doing a study on "language development."[33] For 90 minutes, the children and their parents were recorded doing their regular activities like playing and eating. Everything that was said was then transcribed and analyzed for its content. When these children were between 7 and 8 years old, the same kids completed a questionnaire about their motivations for doing challenging work to help them improve their skills.

The study provided some interesting baseline statistics about praise in young children, such as praise averaging 3% of total parental "utterances" to children. As might be expected, there was *a lot* of variability between families with some parents bestowing 16 times as much praise upon their young children as others. Across all time points, the amount of process praise and person praise was about the same, although person praise tended to become less common relative to process praise as children went from late infancy toward preschool age. Interestingly, most praise reliably could be counted as either process or person oriented, and some consistency was found with regard to how much overall praise a parent gave across time and what type it tended to be. This means you likely have a particular style when it comes to how much you praise and what type of praise you tend to give, even if you haven't been fully aware of that style.

It's good to know this, as understanding your own tendencies when it comes to praise looks to be important. In terms of the main question from the Gunderson study, the researchers found that the children who had received more process praise when very young were more likely years later to like challenging tasks and believe that accomplishments were the result of effort and practice rather than innate abilities. One surprising result that was found, however, was that a parent's own motivational framework didn't seem to match up with the type of praise they uttered. In other words, parents who tended to see success as more a function of effort actually were relatively more likely to use more person praise statements. This finding further supports the possibility that the parents may not be in touch with how to convey their beliefs about motivation to their kids through the types of praise they use (but not anymore, right?). A recent 2017 follow-up of this study when the kids were in fourth grade continued to show these associations between praise type and child attitudes and going further, even demonstrated a link between the amount of process praise given 7 years earlier and higher levels of academic achievement in both reading and math.[34]

Those more skeptical of praise have pointed out that some of these studies can have a hard time disentangling the possibility that what might look like a positive effect of process praise is actually more a negative effect of person praise. Maybe if you just keep quiet and don't really offer praise of any kind, the logic follows, kids will be better off. For example, one study in children from ages 9 to 11 did indicate that simply giving objective feedback for a task, like giving a child their score, was equivalent to giving process praise while giving person praise resulted in a negative effect on a child's feelings and motivation.[35] This study, however, involved the children imagining these different scenarios rather than actually experiencing them and probably isn't enough to warrant tossing away the overall conclusions about process praise. Yet it is also worth pointing out that the main variable of interest in the fairly compelling Gunderson studies was the amount of process praise *relative to total praise*, which leaves open the possibility that part of what may be driving good outcomes relates to giving less overall praise as much as giving more process praise. Countering this critique, however, are other experimental studies that have included a "no praise" group, which have found that process praise is better than no praise at all.[29,36]

This debate brings up the related question of how important it is that a child *consistently* hears process praise. In some of these previously discussed tightly controlled experiments, kids are hearing a short burst of pure process or pure person praise before being evaluated on their performance or motivations, but in the real world children are likely to hear different types of praise throughout the day. How much, then, is your great aunt's wildly inappropriate remark of calling your son a "good boy" going to undermine everyone else's hard work? To get at that, researchers conducted an experimental study in a group of kindergarteners who, similar to some past studies, envisioned themselves drawing things successfully and unsuccessfully and hearing feedback from teachers that had different ratios of process to person praise.[30] They were then asked questions regarding how they felt about themselves (self-evaluation) and about how eager they were to draw something even if it wasn't perfect at first (persistence). What they found was a slightly different pattern for self-evaluation and persistence. For persistence, there was a linear relation between hearing more process praise and feeling more motivated. For self-evaluation, by contrast, hearing even a small proportion of process praise seemed to be helpful. While this study will hardly close the book on the subject on praise consistency, it is somewhat reassuring to hear that a parent doesn't need to impose a gag order on the rest of the world to prevent complete contamination of their efforts to use as much process praise as possible.

Just to make matters more complicated, of course, there is some evidence that things might work a little differently when the outcome being measured is not motivation or achievement but rather being kind and helpful. An older study from 1980 done with 5- to 10-year olds looked at what happened after children were asked to donate some marbles they had "won" in an experiment to less fortunate children. When they did, some were praised for their behavior (e.g., "That was a nice thing to do"), some were praised for their character (e.g., "You must be a nice person"), and some weren't praised at all. When a few weeks later they were again given the opportunity to be generous, the amount kids gave away was found to greatest among those who had been praised for their character, although this finding varied somewhat by age.[37] Some more recent data found similar results. Among a group of 3- to 6-year olds, children were found to be more helpful across different tasks if earlier they had been praised as "a helper" rather than having their specific behavior labeled by an adult as "helping."[38] Looking at dishonest behavior, some of the same researchers found that cheating behavior was significantly less among children who were cautioned not to be "a cheater" compared to being simply asked not to cheat.[39] This inconsistency might suggest that different types of praise works to cultivate different attributes, which could be tough for a parent to keep track of without consulting their notes from moment to moment. Some of this work, however, has been questioned along the lines that person praise might work well with regard to moral behavior when things are going smoothly but is much less stable in the face of the inevitable setbacks.[40] Indeed, one study with 4-year-old children did find that trait-based and specific behavior-based praise are equally reinforcing until someone starts making some mistakes, at which point the kids receiving trait-based person praise act in a more helpless manner.[41] In addition, there is evidence that person praise, when it comes to moral behavior, may lead to more stereotypical beliefs and black-and-white thinking about good versus bad people.[42]

Summing up, the weight of evidence on praise suggests that the type of praise being offered is a very important "it depends" factor and may help explain why there have been so many divergent opinions about the benefits and harms of praise in general. Sincere praise that highlights effort, process, and specific actions have been shown to increase a child's motivation and persistence after a setback or failure, while praise directed at traits such as being smart or being good at something can have the opposite effect and lead children to avoid challenges that might jeopardize their status. This effect has been most intensely studied with regard to a child's motivational level and achievements relative to other areas such as moral actions or levels of emotional-behavioral problems, but at this point there does not seem to be sufficient evidence to recommend vastly different strategies in trying to promote other positive aspects of child development.

Thinking back to Gabrielle and Juanita, the more valid part of the grandfather's criticism may be less about the *amount* of praise Juanita gives her daughter but rather the *type* of praise. Based on the science, Juanita might well want to convert much of her person praise into process praise. She makes a deliberate choice to try it and in the process realizes how automatic she has been with the way she delivers praise. It's not easy, but in so doing she notices that Gabrielle seems to be following her lead and now seem to be more aware herself of the importance of effort and persistence when she does things.

## Remember Process Praise for Girls

In some of the praise studies covered this far, another important factor that arose was gender. In the Gunderson studies, a child's gender didn't seem to change the value of process praise, but the researchers did find that boys tend to hear a higher percentage of process praise compared to girls. The authors linked this finding to other studies that have shown that girls tend to be more likely to attribute failure to lack of ability rather than a lack of effort, which may increase their likelihood to give up after an initial failure.[43] Further, one of the previously described experimental studies with fourth and fifth grade students also showed that the beneficial effects of process praise were present for girls but not boys.[29]

## The Praise Backfire for Kids with Low Self-Esteem

Recall that one of the main motivations for praising children relates to increasing a child's level of self-esteem, especially for those kids who don't already see themselves as valuable, capable, and worthy of attention. While these negative thoughts and feelings can take time to develop, the roots of low self-esteem can certainly be seen and heard in young children as they begin to gain awareness of themselves in relation to others. A child's level of self-esteem is generally not considered to be a stand-alone temperament trait but has been shown to be associated with more established temperament dimensions.[44] In particular, children with lower levels of effortful control and higher levels of negative emotionality, features found in the anxious and agitated temperament types described in chapter 2, may be more likely than other types to struggle with chronic feelings of inadequacy and incompetence.

Trying to help these children feel better about themselves by praising them seems like a natural and effective thing to do, and that is just what many of the official recommendations have been as part of an overall strategy to provide "emotional nourishment" to kids in need.[45] Unfortunately, this extremely well-meaning effort looks like it may actually do more harm than good, particularly if the praise being given is inflated, trait-based, and given for minor things. Studies indicate both that children with lower self-esteem tend to be more likely to be given proportionately more person praise relative to process praise and that such a pattern is associated with these children feeling even more ashamed of themselves after a failure.[46] This interaction can initiate a cycle in which these children end up feeling even worse about themselves, which provokes more person praise, and so on. While such cycles may run against conventional wisdom, this research is beginning to get incorporated even in groups that place great value on the importance of self-esteem such as the National Association for Self-Esteem (http://healthyselfesteem.org), which now states that promoting self-esteem needs to be "tied to reality, not faking reality" and that one cannot increase it by offering "fake praise" to children.

Admittedly, this is some information I wish were not true. Having worked with so many kids who have been made to feel terrible about themselves, it would be so much better if we could just reverse that damage by letting them hear that they are valued and have great potential. In one of my favorite lines from one of my all-time favorite books, *The Cider House Rules* by John Irving,[47] the self-sacrificing doctor running an orphanage in Maine for forgotten and parent-starved children finishes each night by reading them a story and then saying to them, "Good night you princes of Maine, kings of New England." A charter school with predominantly disadvantaged African American students in Nashville, Tennessee, has picked up this tradition by referring to all their students as kings and queens.[48] At this point, I'm not ready to say that the research tells us that we should abandon such practices, but it is fairly clear that much more is required to help these children appreciate their true worth.

## A Critique of Criticism

In my own nonscientific sampling of being around lots of kids and lots of parents at sporting events, birthday parties, and grocery stores, I remain amazed, even in this supposed era of overpraising, at how little adult praise I hear for children relative to the amount of outright scorn, criticism, and name-calling. While my own personal anecdotes shouldn't disqualify the conclusions reached in studies on excessive and misguided praise, I do remain concerned about overpraising as a public health message. In particular, I worry that the mother who frequently calls her young daughter a "little shit" will find the kids are overpraised movement just a little too appealing.

Others agree, and have voiced the opinion that research on the effects of praise cannot be properly understood without also looking simultaneously at how much criticism, especially that which is harsh and mean-spirited, a child receives as well. Child psychologist and author Kenneth Barish writes, when it comes to many demoralized and easily frustrated children, "The culprit is not praise, but criticism. Most of these children were over-criticized, very few were overpraised."[49] Indeed, harsh criticism is one of the indicators of low warmth—a dimension that is characteristic of a more authoritarian parenting style described in chapter 3. In addition to the research summarized there, a vast literature exists on the association between high levels of criticism, often referred to cryptically in the research world as *expressed emotion,* and poor mental health outcomes in both adults and children.[50,51] In 2019, a study of a large sample of children in the United Kingdom found that disciplinary strategies that included shouting and "telling off" children were related to higher levels of emotional problems at age 11.[52]

Despite this evidence, however, we still could use more research that directly investigates the way praise and criticism are related to each other and how effective one really negative comment can be to undermine several positive ones. In the business and management world, there is evidence that the ideal praise to criticism ratio is 5.6 to 1.[53] In 2005, a paper was published in the highly respected journal *American Psychologist* suggesting that, at least for college students, you needed a ratio of three positive emotions to each negative one to help a person "flourish."[54] This study became a bit hit in its ability to calculate one of the essential keys to happiness but later was found to have some faulty math in its methods, which led to the study being discredited. While the field continues to search for that magic ratio, parents may be well advised to keep in mind both sides of the praise/criticism equation.

> Thinking back to Mary and her active deployment of both praise and criticism in her interactions with her son, the problem here may be more related to too much criticism rather than too little praise. Max is already showing signs that the frequency and intensity of his mother's admonishments are exacting a negative toll and could well be sabotaging any positive effects of praise. As Mary begins a conscious effort to reel back the amount of negative comments she makes toward Max, she can see him start to relax more and be less reactive when challenges come his way.

## Putting It All Together

Overall, the scientific data demonstrate pretty convincingly how praising children, as annoying as it may be for some adults to hear, should remain an important part of a parent's toolbox. That said, there are very important "it depends" factors to consider. Praise that is sincere, truly earned, and directed at a child's effort and specific behaviors has been shown to help promote a child's level of persistence and reliance. At the same time, empty and over-the-top praise that focuses on intrinsic traits may actually be worse than no praise at all. This divergence when it comes to the effects of different types of praise may furthermore be particularly prominent among children who suffer from feelings of inadequacy and low self-worth.

The evidence further indicates that some important gender differences may be lurking in the way we give praise to girls versus boys. Girls are relatively more likely to receive person praise that highlights personal characteristics and abilities while boys get a proportionately higher amount of process praise directed at their effort and approach. This discrepancy may partially explain why girls relative to boys tend to attribute failure to a lack of ability rather than a lack of effort—a thought pattern that can lead to giving up prematurely. Finally, another "it depends" factor covered in this chapter relates to the other side of the coin and the frequency and nature of our critical comments to children. We need to remember that the effect of 10 "Good jobs!" might easily get wiped out with one forceful "What's wrong with you!?"

Overall, it is my view that, as a society, we continue to run a praise deficit rather than a surplus. It's a shame that we can't simply transfer some of the superfluous praise bestowed upon very confident children to kids who almost never hear an encouraging word. The trick from a public messaging perspective, it seems, lies in being able to prevent the "too much of a good thing can be harmful" message coming from the research being contorted into a global condemnation of praise itself, ready to be gobbled up by the very people who need to hear this message the least. In saying this, the image that comes to mind is Will Smith's main character in the superhero movie *Hancock* who has to fight every natural inclination in his body to give credit to others and tell them they've done a "g-g-g-g-ood job."

To deliver this message in the most politically effective way, we may be wise to remember that the flip side of the more touchy-feely concept of self-esteem is the much more old school notion of *expectations*. To expect children to meet certain high standards requires believing (and conveying) that they have the capacity to do so. Yet, despite how inextricably linked the two concepts are in practice, somehow the advocacy for praise and self-esteem gets covered by National Public Radio while enforcing high expectations is a subject for Fox News. The lesson here may be to move beyond the politics by understanding that neither principle can stand very well on its own. Lofty demands and expectations are no more likely to succeed in kids who doubt their own value than hollow compliments given to children who lack the necessary tools for success. It is only when appropriate praise is provided in an environment that expects progress and teaches the necessary tools for achievement that a child's full potential as a learner, an artist, or a good friend is fully realized.

## It Depends—Praise

**General Summary**

Praise that is sincere, earned, and directed toward a child's effort and specific behaviors promotes healthy development and achievement and builds motivation to persevere in the face of challenge.

| "It Depends" Factor | Adjustment |
| --- | --- |
| Type of praise | Praise that focuses on specific traits like intelligence or talent can result in *decreased* motivation and perseverance. |
| Gender | Girls are currently more likely to receive praise for traits rather than effort and methods. Parents should actively remember to use process praise for both girls and boys. |
| Self-esteem | Children with negative views of themselves are more sensitive to the negative effects of inflated person praise. |
| Criticism | The positive effects of praise need to be weighed against the negative effects of harsh and frequent criticism. Increasing praise alone without attention to reducing criticism may be ineffective. |

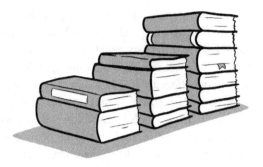

# 13

# The Next Steps

## Putting Knowledge Into Action

If you've made it this far, congratulations! You can now consider yourself to be a truly informed parent when it comes to the topics covered in these chapters. You've heard about a ton of different research studies and hopefully now have a clearer idea about what is really behind some of the most nagging debates in parenting. And while I sincerely hope that the reading process has been enjoyable and am confident that you can robustly hold your ground the next time you find yourself in an online or personal discussion about screens or praise or daycare, many of you probably are asking a very important question right about now.

Now what?

Insight is a crucial and necessary step toward behavior change, but alone it is insufficient. To get all the way to actual changes and improvements in parenting behavior, knowledge needs to be converted into a plan that then gets applied to the routine day-to-day interactions with your children. And unfortunately, as many of you are well aware, it isn't as easy as just saying "Go!"

That is where this chapter comes in. The goal here is to provide some scaffolding and recommendations specifically about *how* you can turn all the new facts and opinions you now have in your brain into something usable for your family. We'll cover skeptical co-parents, prioritization, goal-making, and a relatively simple model that can help you dive into whatever parenting changes you decide to undertake. You can be sure that along the way that things are going to be a little bumpy and you are not going to be perfect. That's okay, because you don't have to be. You can also bet that even when children

Chapter illustrations drawn by Jaq Fagnant

*Parenting Made Complicated.* David C. Rettew, Oxford University Press (2021). © Oxford University Press.
DOI: 10.1093/oso/9780197550977.003.0013

do show benefits from the things you do, the improvements will often not occur quickly. Don't quit. Child development can move like an ocean liner. A lot of momentum has built up getting the boat to go in the direction it is in currently, and steady even pressure is needed to change course *slowly*. As was covered in chapter 3, progress is also more difficult when what needs to happen runs against your own temperamental predispositions, but that is commonly the reality thanks to genetics. Anxious children can have anxious parents, which makes the supportive nudging and exposures that many of these kids need hard for everyone. Children who are prone to lose their temper often have parents with the same challenge. This stacking of the deck is not fair, but it's there nonetheless and is best overcome by both being fully aware of these truths and having a real game plan to help move what *should* be happening to what *is* happening.

## Applying Your Knowledge: Step by Step

In the process of reading these chapters, there likely were many moments when you made little mental bookmarks in your mind—times when a particular behavioral challenge seemed to describe your child to a T or when a proposed recommendation sounded really promising for your own family. Maybe you even took some actual notes. Regardless, it's time now to begin organizing these ideas into a framework that will enable any meaningful change you are hoping for to bear fruit. Before getting into the details, however, you first want to get the other people who parent your child (a spouse, co-parent, nanny, at-home grandparent) involved in the process. "Good luck with that one!" might be your response to that statement. If so, the next section is especially for you.

### The Reluctant Co-Parent

Successful parenting requires there to be a unified front, with everyone involved in caretaking being on the same page, or at least in the same ballpark. If you have identified something in your parenting behavior that you are ready to change, then those of you who are not single parents now need to try to get your spouse, partner, or co-parent aboard. Perhaps you have already tried this by leading a discussion that may have started with "I'm reading this book that talks about (screen time, daycare, etc.), and it suggests that we might want to try . . ." You may have expected some real dialogue to come out of that introduction but instead got a short grunt or perfunctory wave that you fully realize is not going to be enough of a foundation on which to base real change. Maybe you even tried to get your co-parent to read this book or at least a particular chapter, only to get a kind of "I'll get around to it sometime, maybe" response. Now you feel a bit stuck.

First, I'd suggest a little bit of empathy. In addition to leading busy lives, many parents are legitimately skeptical of yet another parenting book by yet another writer telling you how to raise a child the author has never met. You know that this book works a little differently, but *they* don't. To help, I've put together a short invitation letter that you can customize and then encourage your child's co-parent(s) to read in hopes of encouraging more thought, more discussion, and hopefully at some point, more action. Here it is.

---

Dear [insert name here],

[Insert your name here] is in the process of reading this book, entitled *Parenting Made Complicated: What Science Really Knows About the Greatest Debates in Early Childhood*. It's really good and we're hoping that you might take a look too, perhaps reading just a chapter on (a specific topic) as a start. We know you may be a little reluctant to invest your valuable time into reading a parenting book like this. We get that, and we fully understand some of the skepticism you may harbor about parenting books. This one, however, is a little different. It lays out what the science actually says about controversial parenting topics rather than what one author personally thinks is a good idea. It also doesn't pretend that there is a single correct answer for every child and, instead, describes certain characteristics of children, parents, and the environment that might make the best policy for your child at least a little different than for someone else. This book will treat you like a caring, responsible adult, not a heathen needing conversion.

You probably already know how important parenting behavior is to a child's development. Making the right decision for your individual child is not easy and often isn't obvious either. To help, we hope that you might give this book a shot and then discuss what you've read together. [Insert your name here] is very interested in your opinion and in helping your child grow up to be as happy and healthy as possible.

Sincerely,

David Rettew (author of this book) and [insert your name here]

---

To sweeten the pot a little, you may want to consider starting your parenting modifications to target something that is particularly worrisome (or just annoying) to that co-parent. If you have a husband, for example, who is tired of getting elbowed in the face by your toddler every night in bed, maybe the sleep training chapter will pique his interest. If your child's mother yearns for a dinnertime devoid of bribing and threatening your preschooler over eating vegetables, perhaps she will be willing to at least read the section on picky eating. But, if despite your best efforts, your co-parent insists on reading no more than the game scores each day, don't worry! All is not lost, and it is still important and worthwhile to involve him in any discussions about parenting plans or changes, even if the actual parenting modifications need to be done unilaterally, at least in the beginning.

## Start Here

Once the cast has been assembled, the first step is to decide where to focus attention first. For some, this will be an easy choice, and there may be only one or two topics that are even in need of modifications. For others, there might be a temptation to try to fix everything at once and make across-the-board changes on multiple topics covered in these chapters. This approach for most mortals, however, will be extremely challenging and a gradual process is going to feel more manageable for the vast majority of parents.

As an aid in the prioritization sequence, Table 13.1 is designed to provide some key questions to think through on the parenting topics that have been covered in this book.

The first column can help you sort out which parenting topics need any work at all or if they are even applicable to your family at this point. Completing this section will provide an overall view of how many topics will eventually require some attention and what the overall scope of work looks like. From there, you will need to identify in the second column which topics are particularly important to you and most deserving of your first efforts. In some cases, this may be a function of the child's developmental stage. If you are planning for an infant who has yet to be born, for example, then many of the topics can be set as a lower priority simply because they won't be relevant right away. In other instances, however, you may need to make a real choice as to where to focus your efforts. Maybe screen time, discipline, and sleeping are all problematic areas for you and your preschooler. If so, think through which topic or topics are most important right now, keeping in mind that some areas might be highly related to each other, such as discipline and praise. If it is hard to decide, another factor to consider is your level of confidence that you will be able to follow through with your parenting adjustments, as success in one area is likely to enhance the chances of success in another. Finally, you may want to consider undertaking this work, if possible, with the help of a family counselor or therapist who can help you work with the specifics of your own circumstances. Either way, having the list pared down to a topic or two of highest priority will keep this effort from feeling too overwhelming.

Table 13.1 Prioritizing Your Parenting Changes

| Topic | Does the Current Approach to This Topic Need to Change? | How Much of a Priority Is This Particular Subject? (High, Medium, Low) | Initial Goals (Parent and Child if Applicable) |
|---|---|---|---|
| Overall parenting style | | | |
| Childcare arrangements | | | |
| Sleep training | | | |
| Breastfeeding | | | |
| Gender development | | | |
| Eating | | | |
| Divorce and separation | | | |
| Discipline | | | |
| Screens | | | |
| Praise | | | |

The third column is where you will put in some of the initial goals you will have both for yourself and your child. Setting goals sounds easy, but it can be deceptively tricky and can make success more difficult if not done correctly. One commonly used mnemonic for good goal-setting is SMART which stands for making goals that are specific, measurable, attainable, relevant, and time-limited.[1] While some topics lend themselves to SMART goals better than others, these are good criteria to keep in mind. For a toddler who watches 4 hours of screens per day, for example, a more attainable goal may be to reduce it to 2 hours, at least initially, rather than try to stop it completely. You as the parent could also add a goal of doing an extra structured activity together each day, such as reading or going to the park. Goals will be covered in more detail in the next section as part of specific model you can use to operationalize the changes you want to make.

A very reasonable and interesting question at this point has to do with whether or not to engage the child directly in these planning discussions. As you might expect after reading this book, the answer is a resounding *maybe!* with it depending on several factors such as your child's age, maturity level, and anticipated level of resistance to any changes you want to make. Obviously, a preverbal infant won't have much to add to the discussion about how certain clothes may promote gender stereotypes, but a bright preschooler could well contribute to a discussion of which disciplinary strategies are more or less effective. In many cases, involving a child early in the deliberations could improve adherence to any plan that develops as your child is able to take some ownership of that plan.

It also is quite useful before enacting any specific changes to remind yourself what your and your child's temperament is and how that might affect your goals and your plan. Specific instructions for how to do this in a fairly expeditious way can be found in chapter 2. If it has been a while since you did this exercise, now is a good time to refresh your memory. This is important not only to help you choose exactly what type of adjustment you initially want to make to your parenting behavior but to help you anticipate which ones are likely to present smaller or bigger challenges based on your own personality. Maybe, for example, you realize that your 2-year-old's nightly excursion to your bedroom is annoying but that changing this behavior is going to result in a level of conflict that makes you feel anxious and uneasy. Being aware of this obstacle will help you think through strategies that might help you be more successful, such as choosing a sleep training strategy that is likely to provoke less resistance.

## A Model for Improvement

Now that you have everybody on board and have a more focused view of where you want to concentrate your efforts first, the next step is to come up with an actual plan. While it can be quite tempting to avoid these kinds of deliberations for a more spontaneous and less bureaucratic *just do it* mode of implementation, there are reasons to go about this a little more methodically, especially for some of the topics that have been covered in this book. First, it is good to think through exactly what is going to change on your part so that you can best pay attention to how you are doing. Second, keeping in mind the specific and measurable criteria of SMART goals, it's worth articulating what positive change in your child might look like and how you'll know that the new parenting approach is actually having its intended effect. There are lots of ways to define success or failure when it comes to child development, as we have seen from the research studies, and they don't always move in exactly the same direction. A change in approach to your child's picky eating, for example, might result in less conflict at meal times but no discernable improvement in the diversity or amount of food actually being eaten. Is that success? You'll need to decide. Time frames are also an important consideration here as positive change could take a while. A plan to change the way you praise your child, for example, could well improve her level of perseverance and willingness to tackle challenging tasks, but it won't all turn around in a week, or even a month.

One system that has been widely instituted across healthcare facilities trying to do quality improvement work is the Plan–Do–Study–Act (PDSA) model.[2,3] While certainly responsible for a lot of serious eye-rolling among busy doctors who believe that they should be allowed to continue to do things as they always have, the model describes a circular process in which improvements to a system (whether it be a hospital, a doctor's practice, or even the parenting practices of a home) can develop in a systematic and efficient manner. As the name suggests, there are four main components.

- The *Planning* stage in which a specific action plan is designed that includes an assignment for who should do what and predictions about what changes are expected. This also encompasses thoughts about how progress (or lack thereof) will be measured.
- The *Do* stage that actually begins to execute the plan while gathering some data related to the outcomes you are trying to measure. Unexpected problems and variations should also be recorded.
- A *Study* period during which you analyze the data you have gathered to see whether your plan has had the desired effect.
- An *Act* phase (maybe better described as an *Adjust* phase for these purposes) in which modifications to the original plan are discussed. If everything is going great, expansion plans to increase the magnitude or scope of the improvements you've seen can also be considered here.
- Repeat!

Using a PDSA cycle in the context of parenting changes doesn't have to involve a 100-page document or advanced statistical analyses. Here's an example of what this might look like in the context of trying to help a child with picky eating.

George is a 4-year-old boy who has struggled with picky eating for the past year. While he isn't a particularly anxious kid, he's not that adventurous either. After learning more about picky eating and how it might specifically apply to George, his mother, Amy, decides that she is ready to try some changes in the way mealtimes work at home. Her husband, Steve, agrees to try a different approach that they will implement together. Before starting, they agree to follow a PDSA model to help provide some structure to their parenting changes.

*Plan*: Amy and Steve decide in general to implement many of the strategies recommended in the Satter method for a period of 1 month. These will include cutting back on snacks and making a single meal for all family members for lunch and dinner (they decide to continue to allow customized breakfasts at least for now). New foods will be provided to George, but he will not be nagged or incentivized to eat them. Desserts will no longer be dependent on eating "a good dinner" first, although Amy can't bring herself to actually having the dessert served at the same time as the meal. The parents will also try to incorporate George more in the selection and cooking of dinner. Specific outcomes that will be measured at the start and end of the month include (i) his weight, (ii) the level of dinner time conflict and arguing around on a scale of 1 to 10 as rated by all family members, and (iii) the number of new foods he has tried.

*Do:* On a rainy Monday in March, they decide to start. Prior to the first dinner under the new plan, Steve and Amy tell George and his older brother what will be happening. George listens and finds the idea of a noncontingent dessert almost too good to be true but remains somewhat skeptical (they must be up to something). The first dinner is roasted chicken (not breaded), French fries, and green beans. To drink, George asks for juice (an unanticipated development in their plan) and gets it. He eats a few bits of the chicken without protest, and several French fries, while ignoring the green beans. He then declares himself done and heads to the freezer for some ice cream, while George and Amy exchange worried looks. Over the next few weeks, the green beans and other vegetables are repeatedly offered, and one day George nonchalantly puts one in his mouth. At first, the parents enjoy their self-recusal from the role of chief nagger and encourager of eating healthy foods, but as the days continue they find it more and more difficult to hold their tongues.

*Study:* At the end of the month, George has gained 1 pound. The level of conflict at the meal has dropped quite a bit from a score of 8 to a score of 3. While probably a dozen new foods were introduced over the course of the month, George has tried just two of them. Amy and Steve welcome the lack of arguments over meals but think that some modifications are necessary to prod George a bit more, especially now since they are not pushing him to eat the way they used to.

*Act:* The parents introduce a few adjustments to the plan, including the allowance of dessert only three days per week (for the whole family) and limiting juice at mealtimes. George also starts to accompany one of his parents more regularly to the grocery store, where he gets to select some of the fruits and vegetables that the family will eat. With these tweaks based on the experience they have gained over the past month, the family patiently repeats the process and decides to reassess their measures again in one month.

This example demonstrates how a little extra deliberation in the process can provide some much needed structure without demanding extensive amounts of effort or the hiring of a consulting company. The model is well suited for many of the topics covered in this book but particularly for sleep training, praise, screen time, and disciplinary techniques where at least some of the potential benefits of a change in parenting plan can be observed in a relatively short time frame. For others, admittedly, this framework is not as applicable. The potential benefits of breastfeeding, for example, are not going to be seen quickly (with most mothers likely not to be inclined to switch their breastfeeding practices around month to month anyway for the sake of scientific inquiry). These limitations notwithstanding, the PDSA model provides a nice template in which parents can try out the more global recommendations coming out of these chapters for their own children and family.

## Warmth and Positive Energy

In trying to implement the Do and Act phases of this cycle, a critical element that can spell the difference between success and frustration is parental warmth. Recalling back to chapter 3, parental warmth is one of the key elements of the authoritative parenting style, which with some caveats has been shown to be associated with a whole host of good things for children down the road. For many years, I would read research articles describing complex studies that followed kids of all types for many years in the hopes of finding those key factors that would predict long-term happiness and success. What frequently rose to the top wasn't some fancy biological variable like the concentration of serotonin in their cerebrospinal fluid or what medication they took; it was the amount of kindness, affection, and sensitivity a child received from her parents.[4-6] It was parental warmth.

My first reaction was to wave off this "obvious" finding and look for something more interesting to read about, but as it kept coming back, I began to appreciate that parental warmth was something special and precious and not to be taken for granted. Even more, few people were talking about it as a crucial element that it is. And as much as I'd love to impress you right now by telling a story of how I was able to use my own warmth and positive energy to help one of my kids through a challenging situation, not one specific example comes to mind. Fortunately, I can tell you a story about my wife.

Our then 3-year-old son was fairly cautious in nature and often hesitant to try new things. When it was time for his first swim lesson, there was a part of him interested in learning this new skill but also a part that would much rather spend a fun Saturday morning at home. Allowing plenty of extra time, my wife garnered all of her positive energy reserves and, with encouraging statements, jokes, distractions, empathy, and affirmations, proceeded to move him step by step from the house to our gym's swimming pool with our son making outright refusals at *every single turn*. Every proclamation that he would not put on his shoes, get into the car, put on his seatbelt, get out of the car, go into the pool building, take off his shoes, get into the pool, and the like, was met with steady but upbeat reinforcement that he could do this, and that swimming was a fun and worthwhile enterprise. It was truly a parenting masterpiece with her not once going to the dark side and descending into an angry and critical rebuke of our son, which, understandable as it would have been, would have triggered a giant meltdown and destroyed the goal of delivering an emotionally intact child to Cullen, the swim teacher. In the end, we were rewarded with a son who now loves to swim, and this particular morning remains the best example I know of how relentless positive energy can conquer even the most stubborn resistance.

While some people naturally exude warmth and positive emotions (you folks high in extraversion and sociability), these qualities can be tougher to come by for others. Temperamentally, delivering that positive energy for some folks needs to be a force of will, like the summoning of the Petronus Charm in a Harry Potter novel when you least feel happy and optimistic. Warmth and positivity can also be one of the first things to go when a parent is depressed, and this may be one of the pathways through which parental depression can have detrimental effects on child behavior.[7,8] By nature or through thoughtful action, however, the ability to stay positive for as long as possible as you gently try to steer your little ocean liner in a new direction will greatly improve your odds for success.

## And Now—Some More Controversy

It's almost a given that an effort like this book, designed to reduce and explain controversy, will generate some more of its own. Inevitably, there will be many people, some of whom are recognized experts in the field, who will object to even some of the more modest conclusions raised in the previous chapters. Whether it is that the book is too accepting of sleep training, too critical of screen time, too tolerant of time-outs, or too forgiving about divorce, the push back will come. Some will believe that the positions staked out in these pages are extreme, while other will criticize the "wishy washy" stance that the correct parenting decision often is not absolute and depends upon a large number of factors that need to be taken into consideration. Some will maintain that there isn't enough scientific information to draw such firm recommendations, while others will argue that there is *too* much science involved (that can't be trusted anyway due to bias or conflicts of interest). And if you, as a parent or clinician, decide to agree with one or more of the positions described in these chapters and make your view known to others, you can expect some of the same thing.

To all that, I say, *Welcome.* Let's talk! It's a good thing that people get passionate when it comes to parenting because it is indeed a very important topic; the stakes are high for all us. It's also, lest anyone forgot the book's title, quite *complicated* even before all the politics and emotions and personal histories gets layered on top of the science (and many would say also gets baked into the science from the start).

As the parenting debates in cafés, books, social media sites, extended family gatherings, and everywhere else continue, my hope is that all of us can show a willingness to listen to another's sincere viewpoint and show the strength of flexibility either when flaws in our thinking are revealed or when the actual science actually tips the scale in another direction. Remember when all infants were supposed to be put on their stomachs to sleep? Or when carbohydrates were the foundation of a healthy diet? Or when peanuts were to be avoided at all costs for little kids? Recommendations change as science changes, and many parenting controversies, even some that have been with us for a long time, have a database that remains surprisingly small given how common these struggles are and how many headaches they cause. We still are waiting for good randomized studies on strategies for picky eating, better data on what really leads two children with similar gender expressions to diverge on their gender identity, and what the impact of sleep training, if any, is on children with trauma histories. In other areas, the darn topic itself keeps changing, like with screens. Just as we finally approach a consensus about television viewing, kids abandon the medium for something else.

All this may be good news to researchers looking for grant applications or authors hoping to keep writing parenting books, but what about the parents themselves who have to do the best they can with the information they have available right now? You still have to make an initial call based on the science that is out there and then adapt it to the personality of your child and yourself. That call might not be the right one initially, but with a process that allows for judgment-free assessment of how things are going and conscious adjustments along the way, you can slowly move from passively "being a parent" to parenting.

## Some Final Thoughts

Young children are amazing creatures, full of contradictions and inconsistencies. They fall completely apart at the slightest setback yet can show incredible resiliency in the face of major adversity. They absorb qualities of their environment like a sponge, yet can seem driven by internal forces that nothing and no one can alter. They bring parents like us profound joy but also intense worry and, at times, head-banging levels of frustration. But all this is what we signed up for: the sweet sounding laughter, the repeated annoyances, the warm snuggles, and the sleepless nights.

This is the package deal we were offered at the beginning of the trip, and often it feels like the best we can do is hold on and not get thrown off the roller coaster. But if there is any central message to everything you have been reading, it's that this roller coaster is one that you can *steer*, at least enough to get on other pieces of track that hold the promise of a smoother ride. To find those junctions we have the world of parenting science as a guide, which, although complex and changeable, provides at least a solid starting point for decisions to be made. After reading all the information, the conclusions you have drawn about particular topics may vary from my own, but that is fine—the point was never to tell you what to do, but rather to show you what you needed to know and help you appreciate how different kids might need different approaches.

Just the fact that you bothered to read about all these ideas and studies and controversies shows a substantial amount of commitment toward being the best parent that you can. This motivation, coupled with the new knowledge you have gained, can certainly increase your confidence, effectiveness, and (dare I say it) enjoyment as you move though these and other tricky spots in the world of parenting, but it won't completely eliminate either the inevitable missteps or the heartaches associated with them. Thirty years from now, your kids may be talking to a therapist or a close friend about all the blunders and mistakes that you made, but they'll add with a smile about how much you really, really *tried* to do right by them, and, for this journey we call child-raising, that counts for a lot.

# References

## Chapter 1

1. Spock B, Needleman R. *Dr. Spock's Baby and Child Care*. 9th ed. New York, NY: Gallery Books; 2012.

## Chapter 2

1. Chess S, Thomas A. *Temperament in Clinical Practice*. New York, NY: Guilford Press; 1986.
2. Chess S, Thomas A. The New York Longitudinal Study (NYLS): the young adult periods. *Can J Psychiatry*. 1990;35(6):557–561.
3. Rothbart MK. *Becoming Who We Are: Temperament and Personality in Development*. New York, NY: Guilford Press; 2011.
4. Rothbart MK, Ahadi SA, Evans DE. Temperament and personality: origins and outcomes. *J Pers Soc Psychol*. 2000;78(1):122–135.
5. McAdams, TA. *The Art and Science of Personality Development*. New York, NY: Guilford Press; 2015.
6. Kuo PH, Chih YC, Soong WT, Yang HJ, Chen WJ. Assessing personality features and their relations with behavioral problems in adolescents: Tridimensional Personality Questionnaire and Junior Eysenck Personality Questionnaire. *Compr Psychiatry*. 2004;45(1):20–28.
7. Thomas A, Chess S, Birch HG. *Temperament and Behavior Disorders in Children*. New York, NY: New York University Press; 1968.
8. Janson H, Mathiesen KS. Temperament profiles from infancy to middle childhood: development and associations with behavior problems. *Dev Psychol*. 2008;44(5):1314–1328.
9. Kagan J. *Galen's Prophecy*. Boulder, CO: Westview Press; 1994.
10. Rettew DC, Althoff RR, Dumenci L, Ayer L, Hudziak JJ. Latent profiles of temperament and their relations to psychopathology and wellness. *J Am Acad Child Adolesc Psychiatry*. 2008;47(3):273–281.
11. De Clercq B, Rettew D, Althoff RR, De Bolle M. Childhood personality types: vulnerability and adaptation over time. *J Child Psychol Psychiatry*. 2012;53(6):716–722.
12. Rettew DC. *Child Temperament: New Thinking About the Boundary Between Traits and Illness*. New York, NY: W. W. Norton; 2013.
13. Chess S, Thomas A. *Goodness of Fit: Clinical Applications From Infancy Through Adult Life*. Philadelphia, PA: Brunner/Mazel; 1999.
14. Gray J. *Men Are From Mars, Women Are From Venus*. New York, NY: HarperCollins; 1992.
15. Eaton WO. Temperament, development, and the five-factor model: lessons from activity level. In: Halverson CF, Kohnstamm GA, Martin RP, eds. *The Developing*

*Structure of Temperament and Personality From Infancy to Adulthood.* Hillsdale, NJ: Erlbaum; 1994: 173–187.

16. Zahn-Waxler C, Shirtcliff EA, Marceau K. Disorders of childhood and adolescence: gender and psychopathology. *Ann Rev Clin Psychol.* 2008;4:275–303.

17. Saudino KJ. Behavioral genetics and child temperament. *J Dev Behav Pediatr.* 2005;26(3):214–223.

18. Goldsmith HH, Lemery KS, Buss KA, Campos JJ. Genetic analyses of focal aspects of infant temperament. *Dev Psychol.* 1999;35(4):972–985.

19. Rutter M, Dunn J, Plomin R, et al. Integrating nature and nurture: implications of person-environment correlations and interactions for developmental psychopathology. *Dev Psychopathology.* 1997;9(2):335–364.

20. Klein MR, Lengua LJ, Thompson SF, et al. Bidirectional relations between temperament and parenting predicting preschool-age children's adjustment. *J Clin Child Adolesc Psychol.* 2018;47(Supp 1):S113–S126.

21. DiLalla LF, Jones S. Genetic and environmental influences on temperament in preschoolers. In: Molfese VJ, Molfese DL, eds. *Temperament and Personality Development Across the Life Span.* Mahway, NJ: Erlbaum; 2000: 33–55.

22. Champagne FA, McCabe A. Genes in context: gene-environment interplay and the origins of individual differences in behavior. *Curr Direct Psychol Science.* 2013;18:127–131.

23. Ivorra JL, Sanjuan J, Jover M, Carot JM, Frutos R, Molto MD. Gene–environment interaction of child temperament. *J Dev Behav Pediatr.* 2010;31(7):545–554.

24. Kochanska G, Philibert RA, Barry RA. Interplay of genes and early mother-child relationship in the development of self-regulation from toddler to preschool age. *J Child Psychol Psychiatry.* 2009;50(11):1331–1338.

25. McGowan PO, Sasaki A, D'Alessio AC, et al. Epigenetic regulation of the glucocorticoid receptor in human brain associates with childhood abuse. *Nat Neurosci.* 2009;12(3):342–348.

26. Slagt M, Dubas JS, Dekovic M, van Aken MA. Differences in sensitivity to parenting depending on child temperament: a meta-analysis. *Psychol Bull.* 2016;142(10):1068–1110.

## Chapter 3

1. Sax L. *The Collapse of Parenting: How We Hurt Our Kids When We Treat Them Like Grown-Ups.* New York, NY: Basic Books; 2015.

2. Hoefle V, Kajitani A. *Duct Tape Parenting: A Less Is More Approach to Raising Respectful, Responsible, and Resilient Kids.* New York, NY: Bibliomotion; 2012.

3. Chua A. *Battle Hymn of the Tiger Mother.* London, UK: Bloomsbury; 2011.

4. Doephke M, Zilibotti F. *Love, Money & Parenting: How Economics Explains the Way We Raise Our Kids.* Princeton, NJ: Princeton University Press; 2019.

5. Ishizuka P. Social class, gender, and contemporary parenting standards in the United States: evidence from a national survey experiment. *Soc Forces.* 2019;98(1):31–58.

6. Ainsworth MS, Blehar MC, Waters E, Wall S. *Patterns of Attachment: A Psychological Study of the Strange Situation.* Hillsdale, NJ: Erlbaum; 1978.

7. Fearon RP, Bakermans-Kranenburg MJ, van Ijzendoorn MH, Lapsley AM, Roisman GI. The significance of insecure attachment and disorganization in the

development of children's externalizing behavior: a meta-analytic study. *Child Dev.* 2010;81(2):435–456.

8. Sroufe B. The role of infant-caregiver attachment in development. In: Belsky J, Nezworski T, eds. *Clinical Implications of Attachment.* Hillsdale, NJ: Erlbaum; 1988:18–40.

9. Rettew DC, McKee L. Temperament and its role in developmental psychopathology. *Harvard Rev Psychiat.* 2005;13(1):14–27.

10. Sears B, Sears M. *The Attachment Parenting Book: A Commonsense Guide to Understanding and Nurturing Your Baby.* Boston, MA: Little, Brown; 2001.

11. Sears W, Sears M. Attachment parenting babies are raised the way nature intended. *Ask Dr. Sears.* https://www.askdrsears.com/topics/parenting/attachment-parenting/attachment-parenting-babies. Accessed October 9, 2017.

12. Nicholson B, Parker L. *Attached to the Heart: Eight Proven Parenting Principles for Raising Connected and Compassionate Children.* Deerfield Beach, FL: Health Communications; 2013.

13. Kim SY, Wang Y, Orozco-Lapray D, Shen Y, Murtuza M. Does "tiger parenting" exist? Parenting profiles of Chinese Americans and adolescent developmental outcomes. *Asian Am J Psychol.* 2013;4(1):7–18.

14. Kang S. *The Dolphin Way: A Parent's Guide to Raising Happy, Healthy, and Motivated Kids—Without Turning Into a Tiger.* New York, NY: Penguin Random House; 2014.

15. Duckworth A. *Grit: The Power of Passion and Perseverance* New York, NY: Scribner; 2016.

16. Skenazy L. *Free-Range Kids: Giving Our Children the Freedom We Had Without Going Nuts With Worry.* San Francisco, CA: Jossey-Bass; 2009.

17. Flynn M. Utah's "free-range parenting" law said to be first in the nation. *Washington Post.* March 28, 2018.

18. Baumrind D. The influence of parenting style on adolescent competence and substance use. *J Early Adolesc.* 1991;11:56–95.

19. Maccoby EE, Martin JA. Socialization in the context of the family: parent–child interaction. In: Mussen PH, ed. *Handbook of Child Psychology.* Vol 4. 4th ed. New York: Wiley; 1983:1–101.

20. The collapse of parenting: how we hurt our kids when we treat them like grown-ups. *Publishers Weekly.* 2015;262:72.

21. Moyer MW. There has been no collapse of parenting. *Slate.* Published Jan 22, 2016. https://slate.com/human-interest/2016/01/leonard-sax-is-wrong-authoritarian-parenting-can-be-bad-for-kids.html

22. Skenazy L. "Helicopter parenting works," say New York Times. But—. LetGrow.org. Published May 13, 2019.

23. DeVore ER, Ginsburg K. The protective effects of good parenting on adolescents. *Curr Opin Pediatr.* 2005;17(4):460–465.

24. Pinquart M. Associations of parenting dimensions and styles with externalizing problems of children and adolescents: an updated meta-analysis. *Dev Psychol.* 2017;53(5):873–932.

25. Steinberg L, Blatt-Eisengart I, Cauffman E. Patterns of competence and adjustment among adolescents from authoritative, authoritarian, indulgent, and neglectful homes: a replication in a sample of serious juvenile offenders. *J Res Adolesc.* 2006;16(1):47–58.

26. Berge J, Sundell K, Ojehagen A, Hakansson A. Role of parenting styles in adolescent substance use: results from a Swedish longitudinal cohort study. *BMJ Open.* 2016;6(1):e008979.

27. Baumrind D. Rejoinder to Lewis' reinterpretation of parental firm control effects: are authoritative families really harmonious? *Psychol Bull.* 1983;94:132–142.

28. Querido JG, Warner TD, Eyberg SM. Parenting styles and child behavior in African American families of preschool children. *J Clin Child Adolesc Psychol.* 2002;31(2):272–277.

29. Whittle S, Vijayakumar N, Simmons JG, et al. Role of positive parenting in the association between neighborhood social disadvantage and brain development across adolescence. *JAMA Psychiatry.* 2017;74(8):824–832.

30. Buri J. Parental authority questionnaire. *J Pers Assess.* 1991;57(1):110–119.

31. Mebust K, Rettew DC, Hudziak JJ. *Effect of ADHD on Parenting: Evidence for an Evocative Gene–Environment Correlation.* Paper presented at the 57th Annual Meeting of the American Academy of Child and Adolescent Psychiatry, February, 2010; New York, NY.

32. Smetana JG. Current research on parenting styles, dimensions, and beliefs. *Curr Opin Psychol.* 2017;15:19–25.

33. Pinquart M, Kauser R. Do the associations of parenting styles with behavior problems and academic achievement vary by culture? Results from a meta-analysis. *Cultur Divers Ethnic Minor Psychol.* 2018;24(1):75–100.

34. Garcia F, Gracia E. Is always authoritative the optimum parenting style? Evidence from Spanish families. *Adolescence.* 2009;44(173):101–131.

35. Slagt M, Dubas JS, Dekovic M, van Aken MA. Differences in sensitivity to parenting depending on child temperament: a meta-analysis. *Psychol Bull.* 2016;142(10):1068–1110.

36. Pluess M, Belsky J. Differential susceptibility to parenting and quality child care. *Dev Psychol.* 2010;46(2):379–390.

37. Williams LR, Degnan KA, Perez-Edgar KE, et al. Impact of behavioral inhibition and parenting style on internalizing and externalizing problems from early childhood through adolescence. *J Abnorm Child Psychol.* 2009;37(8):1063–1075.

38. Mills RSL, Rubin KH. Socialization factors in the development of social withdrawal. In: Rubin KH, Asendorpf J, eds. *Social Withdrawal, Inhibition, and Shyness in Childhood.* Hillsdale, NJ: Erlbaum; 1993:117–148.

39. Van Leeuwen KG, Mervielde I, Braet C, Bosmans G. Child personality and parental behavior as moderators of problem behavior: variable- and person-centered approaches. *Dev Psychol.* 2004;40(6):1028–1046.

40. Kochanska G. Socialization and temperament in the development of guilt and conscience. *Child Dev.* 1991;62(1379–1392).

41. Cornell AH, Frick PJ. The moderating effects of parenting styles in the association between behavioral inhibition and parent-reported guilt and empathy in preschool children. *J Clin Child Adolesc Psychol.* 2007;36(3):305–318.

# Chapter 4

1. Banks S, Dinges DF. Behavioral and physiological consequences of sleep restriction. *J Clin Sleep Med.* 2007;3(5):519–528.

2. Medina AM, Lederhos CL, Lillis TA. Sleep disruption and decline in marital satisfaction across the transition to parenthood. *J Collab Family Healthc.* 2009;27(2):153–160.

3. Sadeh A, Gruber R, Raviv A. Sleep, neurobehavioral functioning, and behavior problems in school-age children. *Child Dev.* 2002;73(2):405–417.

4. Dennis CL, Ross L. Relationships among infant sleep patterns, maternal fatigue, and development of depressive symptomatology. *Birth*. 2005;32(3):187–193.

5. Mindell JA, Kuhn B, Lewin DS, Meltzer LJ, Sadeh A. Behavioral treatment of bedtime problems and night wakings in infants and young children. *Sleep*. 2006;29(10):1263–1276.

6. Mindell JA, Owens JA. *Clinical Guide to Pediatric Sleep: Diagnosis and Management of Sleep Problems*. Philadelphia, PA: Lippincott Williams & Wilkins; 2003.

7. Thomas A, Chess S, Birch HG, Hertzig ME, Korn S. *Behavioral Individuality in Early Childhood*. New York, NY: New York University Press; 1963.

8. Fisher A, van Jaarsveld CH, Llewellyn CH, Wardle J. Genetic and environmental influences on infant sleep. *Pediatrics*. 2012;129(6):1091–1096.

9. Brescianini S, Volzone A, Fagnani C, et al. Genetic and environmental factors shape infant sleep patterns: a study of 18-month-old twins. *Pediatrics*. 2011;127(5):e1296–1302.

10. Touchette E, Dionne G, Forget-Dubois N, et al. Genetic and environmental influences on daytime and nighttime sleep duration in early childhood. *Pediatrics*. 2013;131(6):e1874–1880.

11. France KG, Blampied NM. Infant sleep disturbance: description of a problem behaviour process. *Sleep Med Rev*. 1999;3(4):265–280.

12. Sears W, Sears M. Attachment parenting babies are raised the way nature intended. *Ask Dr. Sears*. https://www.askdrsears.com/topics/parenting/attachment-parenting/attachment-parenting-babies. Accessed October 9, 2017.

13. Holt LE. *Care and Feeding of Children: A Catechism for the Use of Mother's and Children's Nurses*. New York, NY: D. Appleton; 1906.

14. Williams CD. The elimination of tantrum behavior by extinction procedures. *J Abnorm Soc Psychology*. 1959;59:269.

15. Ferber R. *Solve Your Child's Sleep Problems*. New York, NY: Fireside; 2006.

16. Rolider A, Van Houten R. Training parents to use extinction to eliminate nighttime crying by gradually increasing the criteria for ignoring crying. *Educ Treat Child*. 1984;7:119–124.

17. Seabrook J. Sleeping with the baby. *The New Yorker*. https://www.newyorker.com/magazine/1999/11/08/sleeping-with-the-baby. Published November 8, 1999.

18. Barajas RG, Martin A, Brooks-Gunn J, Hale L. Mother–child bed-sharing in toddlerhood and cognitive and behavioral outcomes. *Pediatrics*. 2011;128(2):e339–e347.

19. Matthey S, Crncec R. Comparison of two strategies to improve infant sleep problems, and associated impacts on maternal experience, mood and infant emotional health: a single case replication design study. *Early Hum Dev*. 2012;88(6):437–442.

20. Milan MA, Mitchell ZP, Berger MI, Pierson DF. Positive routines: a rapid alternative to extinction for elimination of bedtime tantrum behavior. *Child Beh Ther*. 1981;3:13–25.

21. Gradisar M, Jackson K, Spurrier NJ, et al. Behavioral interventions for infant sleep problems: a randomized controlled trial. *Pediatrics*. 2016;137(6). e20151486.

22. Haelle T, Willingham E. *The Informed Parent: A Science-Based Resource for Your Child's First Four Years*. New York, NY: TarcherPerigee; 2016.

23. Bartick M, Smith LJ. Speaking out on safe sleep: evidence-based infant sleep recommendations. *Breastfeed Med*. 2014;9(9):417–422.

24. Gao Y, Schwebel DC, Hu G. Infant mortality due to unintentional suffocation among infants younger than 1 year in the United States, 1999-2015. *JAMA Pediatrics*. 2018;172(4):388–390.

25. Vennemann MM, Hense HW, Bajanowski T, et al. Bed sharing and the risk of sudden infant death syndrome: can we resolve the debate? *J Pediatrics*. 2012;160(1):44–48 e42.

26. Carpenter R, McGarvey C, Mitchell EA, et al. Bed sharing when parents do not smoke: is there a risk of SIDS? An individual level analysis of five major case-control studies. *BMJ Open*. 2013;3(5).

27. Blabey MH, Gessner BD. Infant bed-sharing practices and associated risk factors among births and infant deaths in Alaska. *Pub Health Rep*. 2009;124(4):527–534.

28. Blair PS, Sidebotham P, Pease A, Fleming PJ. Bed-sharing in the absence of hazardous circumstances: is there a risk of sudden infant death syndrome? An analysis from two case-control studies conducted in the UK. *PLoS One*. 2014;9(9):e107799.

29. Hiscock H, Bayer J, Gold L, Hampton A, Ukoumunne OC, Wake M. Improving infant sleep and maternal mental health: a cluster randomised trial. *Arch Dis Childhood*. 2007;92(11):952–958.

30. Hiscock H, Bayer JK, Hampton A, Ukoumunne OC, Wake M. Long-term mother and child mental health effects of a population-based infant sleep intervention: cluster-randomized, controlled trial. *Pediatrics*. 2008;122(3):e621–627.

31. Price AM, Wake M, Ukoumunne OC, Hiscock H. Five-year follow-up of harms and benefits of behavioral infant sleep intervention: randomized trial. *Pediatrics*. 2012;130(4):643–651.

32. Narvaez D. Dangers of "crying it out". *Psychology Today*. https://www.psychologytoday.com/us/blog/moral-landscapes/201112/dangers-crying-it-out. Published December 11, 2011.

# Chapter 5

1. Belsky J. Emanuel Miller lecture: developmental risks (still) associated with early child care. *J Child Psychol Psychiatry*. 2001;42(7):845–859.

2. US Department of Labor, Bureau of Labor Statistics. Employment characteristics of families—2017. http://www.bls.gov/news.release/pdf/famee.pdf. Accessed July 3, 2018.

3. Belsky J, Vandell DL, Burchinal M, et al. Are there long-term effects of early child care? *Child Dev*. 2007;78(2):681–701.

4. Donnelly K, Twenge JM, Clark MA, Shaikh SK, Beiler-May A, Carter NT. Attitudes toward women's work and family roles in the United States, 1976–2013. *Women's Res Q*. 2016;40(1):41–54.

5. Hijat M. Can affectional ties be purchased? Comments on working mothers and their families. *J Soc Behav Pers*. 1990;5:493–502.

6. Leach P. *Children First: What Our Society Must Do—and Is Doing—for Our Children Today*. New York NY: Oxford University Press; 1994.

7. Belsky J. Infant day care: a cause for concern? *Zero to Three*. 1986;7(1):1–7.

8. Gentleman A. The great nursery debate. *The Guardian*. https://www.theguardian.com/lifeandstyle/2010/oct/02/nurseries-childcare-pre-school-cortisol. Published October 1, 2010.

9. NICHD Early Child Care Research Network. *Child Care and Child Development: Results From the NICHD Study of Early Child Care and Youth Development*. New York, NY: Guilford Press; 2005.

10. NICHD Early Child Care Research Network. Early child care and children's development in the primary grades: results from the NICHD study of early child care. *Am Educ Res Jl.* 2005;43:537–570.

11. NICHD Early Child Care Research Network. Child-care effect sizes for the NICHD study of early child care and youth development. *Am Psychologist.* 2006;61(2):99–116.

12. NICHD Early Child Care Research Network. Does amount of time spent in child care predict socioemotional adjustment during the transition to kindergarten? *Child Dev.* 2003;74(4):976–1005.

13. Crockenberg SC. Rescuing the baby from the bathwater: how gender and temperament (may) influence how child care affects child development. *Child Dev.* 2003;74(4):1034–1038.

14. Belsky J. Quantity counts: amount of child care and children's socioemotional development. *J Dev Behav Pediatr.* 2002;23(3):167–170.

15. NICHD Early Child Care Research Network. Type of child care and children's development at 54 months. *Early Child Res Q.* 2004;19:203–230.

16. Belsky J, Rovine M. Nonmaternal care in the first year of life and security of infant-parent attachment. *Child Dev.* 1988;59:157–167.

17. NICHD Early Child Care Research Network. The effects of infant child care on infant-mother attachment security: results of the NICHD study of early child care *Child Dev.* 1997;68(5):860–879.

18. Hagekull B, Bohlin G. Day care quality, family and child characteristics and socioemotional development. *Early Child Res Q.* 1995;10:505–526.

19. Vandell DL, Belsky J, Burchinal M, Steinberg L, Vandergrift N. Do effects of early child care extend to age 15 years? Results from the NICHD study of early child care and youth development. *Child Dev.* 2010;81(3):737–756.

20. Sweeney JF. Jay Belsky doesn't play well with others. *Salon.* https://www.salon.com/2001/04/26/belsky. Published April 26, 2001.

21. Ballance BA. 7 reasons to feel empowered as a working mom. *Babble.* https://www.psychologytoday.com/us/articles/200505/the-trouble-day-care. Published February 13, 2018.

22. Lang H. The trouble with daycare. *Psychology Today.* https://www.psychologytoday.com/us/articles/200505/the-trouble-day-care. Updated June 9, 2015.

23. Sammons P, Elliot K, Sylva K, Melhuish E, Siraj-Blatchford I, Taggert B. The impact of pre-school on young children's cognitive attainments at entry to reception. *Brit Educ Res J.* 2004;30(5):691–712.

24. Lucas-Thompson RG, Goldberg WA, Prause J. Maternal work early in the lives of children and its distal associations with achievement and behavior problems: a meta-analysis. *Psychol Bull.* 2010;136(6):915–942.

25. McGinn KL, Castro MR, Lingo EL. Learning from mum: cross-national evidence linking maternal employment and adult children's outcomes. *Work Employ Society.* 2019;33(3):374–400.

26. National Institute of Child Health and Human Development. *The NICHD study of early child care and youth development: Findings for children up to 4 1/2 years.* NIH Pub 05-4318, 2006. https://www.nichd.nih.gov/sites/default/files/publications/pubs/documents/seccyd_06.pdf. Published 2006.

27. Reynolds A. *Success in Early Childhood Interventions: The Chicago Child–Parent Centers.* Lincoln, NE: University of Nebraska; 2000.

28. Campbell FA, Pungello EP, Miller-Johnson S, Burchinal M, Ramey C. The development of cognitive and academic abilities: growth curves from an early intervention educational experiment. *Dev Psychology*. 2001;37:231–242.
29. Howes C, Olenick M. Family and child care influences on toddlers' compliance. *Child Dev*. 1986;57:202–216.
30. Egeland B, Heister M. The long-term consequences of infant day-care and mother–infant attachment. *Child Dev*. 1995;66:74–85.
31. Fox NA, Henderson HA, Marshall PJ, Nichols KE, Ghera MM. Behavioral inhibition: linking biology and behavior within a developmental framework. *Ann Rev Psychology*. 2005;56:235–262.
32. Pluess M, Belsky J. Prenatal programming of postnatal plasticity? *Dev Psychopathology*. 2011;23(1):29–38.
33. Pluess M, Belsky J. Differential susceptibility to parenting and quality child care. *Dev Psychol*. 2010;46(2):379–390.
34. Slagt M, Dubas JS, Dekovic M, van Aken MA. Differences in sensitivity to parenting depending on child temperament: a meta-analysis. *Psychol Bull*. 2016;142(10):1068–1110.
35. Dettling AC, Gunnar MR, Donzella B. Cortisol levels of young children in full-day childcare centers: relations with age and temperament. *Psychoneuroendocrinology*. 1999;24(5):519–536.
36. Dettling AC, Parker SW, Lane S, Sebanc A, Gunnar MR. Quality of care and temperament determine changes in cortisol concentrations over the day for young children in childcare. *Psychoneuroendocrinology*. 2000;25(8):819–836.
37. Vermeer HJ, van IJzendoorn MH. Children's elevated cortisol levels at daycare: a review and meta-analysis. *Early Child Res Q*. 2006;21(3):390–401.
38. Fox NA, Henderson HA, Rubin KH, Calkins SD, Schmidt LA. Continuity and discontinuity of behavioral inhibition and exuberance: psychophysiological and behavioral influences across the first four years of life. *Child Dev*. 2001;72(1):1–21.
39. Degnan KA, Henderson HA, Fox NA, Rubin KH. Predicting social wariness in middle childhood: the moderating roles of child care history, maternal personality and maternal behavior. *Soc Dev*. 2008;17(3):471–487.

## Chapter 6

1. Callahan A. *The Science of Mom: A Research-Based Guide to Your Baby's First Year*. Baltimore, MD: John Hopkins University Press; 2015.
2. Jung C. *Lactivism*. Philadelphia, PA: Basic Books; 2015.
3. Centers for Disease Control and Prevention. Breastfeeding report card—United States, 2018. https://www.cdc.gov/breastfeeding/data/reportcard.htm. Published August 20, 2018.
4. American Academy of Pediatrics. Breastfeeding and the use of human milk. *Pediatrics*. 2012;129(3):e827–e841.
5. Bartick M, Reinhold A. The burden of suboptimal breastfeeding in the United States: a pediatric cost analysis. *Pediatrics*. 2010;125(5):e1048–1056.
6. Victora CG, Horta BL, Loret de Mola C, et al. Association between breastfeeding and intelligence, educational attainment, and income at 30 years of age: a prospective birth cohort study from brazil. *Lancet Glob Health*. 2015;3(4):e199–205.

7. Angelsen NK, Vik T, Jacobsen G, Bakketeig LS. Breast feeding and cognitive development at age 1 and 5 years. *Arch Dis Childhood*. 2001;85(3):183–188.

8. Der G, Batty GD, Deary IJ. Effect of breast feeding on intelligence in children: prospective study, sibling pairs analysis, and meta-analysis. *BMJ*. 2006;333(7575):945.

9. Anderson JW, Johnstone BM, Remley DT. Breast-feeding and cognitive development: a meta-analysis. *Am J Clin Nutrition*. 1999;70(4):525–535.

10. Ip S, Chung M, Raman G, et al. Breastfeeding and maternal and infant health outcomes in developed countries. *Evid Rep Technol Assess*. 2007(153):1–186.

11. Lucas A, Morley R, Cole TJ, Lister G, Leeson-Payne C. Breast milk and subsequent intelligence quotient in children born preterm. *Lancet*. 1992;339(8788):261–264.

12. Morrow-Tlucak M, Haude RH, Ernhart CB. Breastfeeding and cognitive development in the first 2 years of life. *Soc Sci Med*. 1988;26(6):635–639.

13. Girard LC, Doyle O, Tremblay RE. Breastfeeding, cognitive and noncognitive development in early childhood: a population study. *Pediatrics*. 2017;139(4):e 20161848.

14. Bernard JY, Armand M, Peyre H, et al. Breastfeeding, polyunsaturated fatty acid levels in colostrum and child intelligence quotient at age 5–6 years. *J Pediatrics*. 2017;183:43–50.

15. Andres A, Cleves MA, Bellando JB, Pivik RT, Casey PH, Badger TM. Developmental status of 1-year-old infants fed breast milk, cow's milk formula, or soy formula. *Pediatrics*. 2012;129(6):1134–1140.

16. Belfort MB, Rifas-Shiman SL, Kleinman KP, et al. Infant feeding and childhood cognition at ages 3 and 7 years: effects of breastfeeding duration and exclusivity. *JAMA Pediatrics*. 2013;167(9):836–844.

17. Jacobson SW, Chiodo LM, Jacobson JL. Breastfeeding effects on intelligence quotient in 4- and 11-year-old children. *Pediatrics*. 1999;103(5):e71.

18. Wigg NR, Tong S, McMichael AJ, Baghurst PA, Vimpani G, Roberts R. Does breastfeeding at six months predict cognitive development? *Austral NZ J Pub Health*. 1998;22(2):232–236.

19. Horta BL, Loret de Mola C, Victora CG. Breastfeeding and intelligence: a systematic review and meta-analysis. *Acta Paediatr*. 2015;104(467):14–19.

20. Kramer MS, Aboud F, Mironova E, et al. Breastfeeding and child cognitive development: new evidence from a large randomized trial. *Arch Gen Psychiatry*. 2008;65(5):578–584.

21. Kramer MS, Fombonne E, Igumnov S, et al. Effects of prolonged and exclusive breastfeeding on child behavior and maternal adjustment: evidence from a large, randomized trial. *Pediatrics*. 2008;121(3):e435–440.

22. Der G, Batty GD, Deary IJ. Results from the PROBIT breastfeeding trial may have been overinterpreted. *Arch Gen Psychiatry*. 2008;65(12):1456–1457; author reply 1458–1459.

23. Evenhouse E, Reilly S. Improved estimates of the benefits of breastfeeding using sibling comparisons to reduce selection bias. *Health Serv Res*. 2005;40(6 Pt 1):1781–1802.

24. Das UN, Fams. Long-chain polyunsaturated fatty acids in the growth and development of the brain and memory. *Nutrition*. 2003;19(1):62–65.

25. Marszalek JR, Lodish HF. Docosahexaenoic acid, fatty acid-interacting proteins, and neuronal function: breastmilk and fish are good for you. *Annu Rev Cell Dev Biol*. 2005;21:633–657.

26. Herba CM, Roza S, Govaert P, et al. Breastfeeding and early brain development: the Generation R study. *Matern Child Nutr*. 2013;9(3):332–349.

27. Isaacs EB, Fischl BR, Quinn BT, Chong WK, Gadian DG, Lucas A. Impact of breast milk on intelligence quotient, brain size, and white matter development. *Pediatr Res.* 2010;67(4):357–362.

28. Caspi A, Williams B, Kim-Cohen J, et al. Moderation of breastfeeding effects on the IQ by genetic variation in fatty acid metabolism. *Proc Natl Acad Sci U S A.* 2007;104(47):18860–18865.

29. Oken E, Radesky JS, Wright RO, et al. Maternal fish intake during pregnancy, blood mercury levels, and child cognition at age 3 years in a us cohort. *Am J Epidemiology.* 2008;167(10):1171–1181.

30. Luby JL, Belden AC, Whalen D, Harms MP, Barch DM. Breastfeeding and childhood IQ: the mediating role of gray matter volume. *J Am Acad Child Adolesc Psychiatry.* 2016;55(5):367–375.

31. Weaver IC, Cervoni N, Champagne FA, et al. Epigenetic programming by maternal behavior. *Nat Neurosci.* 2004;7(8):847–854.

32. Belfort MB, Anderson PJ, Nowak VA, et al. Breast milk feeding, brain development, and neurocognitive outcomes: a 7-year longitudinal study in infants born at less than 30 weeks' gestation. *J Pediatrics.* 2016;177:133–139.e1.

33. Brion MJ, Lawlor DA, Matijasevich A, et al. What are the causal effects of breastfeeding on IQ, obesity and blood pressure? Evidence from comparing high-income with middle-income cohorts. *Int J Epidemiology.* 2011;40(3):670–680.

34. Koh K. Maternal breastfeeding and children's cognitive development. *Soc Sci Med.* 2017;187:101–108.

# Chapter 7

1. Servin AGG, Berlin L. Sex differences in 1-, 3-. and 5-year-olds' toy-choice in a structured play session. *Scand J Psychology.* 1999;40:43–48.

2. van de Beek CSH, van Goozen SH, Buitelaar JK, Cohen-Kettenis PT. Prenatal sex hormones (maternal and amniotic fluid) and gender-related play behavior in 13-month-old infants. *Arch Sex Behavior.* 2009;38:6–15.

3. Maccoby EE. *The Two Sexes: Growing Up Apart, Coming Together.* Cambridge, MA: Harvard University Press; 1998.

4. Eliot L. *Pink Brain, Blue Brain: How Small Differences Grow Into Troublesome Gaps— and What We Can Do About It.* New York: Houghton Mifflin Harcourt; 2009.

5. GLAAD. [Home page]. https://www.glaad.org/. Accessed October 4, 2018.

6. Ngun TC, Ghahramani N, Sanchez FJ, Bocklandt S, Vilain E. The genetics of sex differences in brain and behavior. *Front Neuroendocrinol.* 2011;32(2):227–246.

7. Bao AM, Swaab DF. Sexual differentiation of the human brain: relation to gender identity, sexual orientation and neuropsychiatric disorders. *Front Neuroendocrinol.* 2011;32(2):214–226.

8. Iervolino AC, Hines M, Golombok SE, Rust J, Plomin R. Genetic and environmental influences on sex-typed behavior during the preschool years. *Child Dev.* 2005;76(4):826–840.

9. Colapinto J. *As Nature Made Him: The Boy Who Was Raised as a Girl.* New York, NY: Harper Collins; 2006.

10. Meyer-Bahlburg HF. Gender identity outcome in female-raised 46,XY persons with penile agenesis, cloacal exstrophy of the bladder, or penile ablation. *Arch Sex Behav.* 2005;34(4):423–438.

11. Berenbaum SA, Beltz AM, Bryk K, McHale S. Gendered peer involvement in girls with congenital adrenal hyperplasia: effects of prenatal androgens, gendered activities, and gender cognitions. *Arch Sex Behav*. 2018;47(4):915–929.

12. Emanuel D. Raising an intersex child: "This is your body. . . . There's nothing to be ashamed of." https://www.cnn.com/2019/04/13/health/intersex-child-parenting-eprise/index.html. Published April 15, 2019.

13. Loehlin JC, Martin NG. Dimensions of psychological masculinity–femininity in adult twins from opposite-sex and same-sex pairs. *Behav Genet*. 2000;30(1):19–28.

14. Alexander GM, Wilcox T, Woods R. Sex differences in infants' visual interest in toys. *Arch Sex Behav*. 2009;38(3):427–433.

15. Hassett JM, Siebert ER, Wallen K. Sex differences in rhesus monkey toy preferences parallel those of children. *Horm Behav*. 2008;54:348–364.

16. Joel D, Berman Z, Tavor I, et al. Sex beyond the genitalia: the human brain mosaic. *Proc Natl Acad Sci U S A*. 2015;112(50):15468–15473.

17. Bakker J. *Brain Structure and Function in Gender Dysphoria*. Paper presented at the 20th European Conference of Endocrinology, 2018; Barcelona, Spain.

18. Blum RW, Mmari K, Moreau C. It begins at 10: how gender expectations shape early adolescence around the world. *J Adolesc Health*. 2017;61(4S):S3–S4.

19. Saewyc E. A global perspective on gender roles and identity. *J Adolesc Health*. 2017;61(4S):S1–S2.

20. World Economic Forum. The global gender gap report 2017. https://www.weforum.org/reports/the-global-gender-gap-report-2017. Published November 2, 2017.

21. Henderson BA, Berenbaum SA. Sex-typed play in opposite-sex twins. *Dev Psychobiol*. 1997;31(2):115–123.

22. Serbin LA, Conner JM, Burchardt CJ, Citron CC. Effects of peer presence on sex-typing of children's play behavior. *J Exper Child Psychology*. 1979;27:303–309.

23. Haviland JJ, Malatesta CZ. The development of sex differences in nonverbal signals: Fallacies, fact, and fantasies. In: Mayo C, Henley NM, eds. *Gender and Nonverbal Behavior*. New York: Springer-Verlag; 1981: 183–208.

24. Stern M, Karraker KH. Sex stereotyping of infants: a review of gender labeling studies. *Sex Roles*. 1989;20:501–522.

25. Quinn PC, Yahr J, Kuhn A, Slater AM, Pascalils O. Representation of the gender of human faces by infants: a preference for female. *Perception*. 2002;31(9):1109–1121.

26. Lytton H, Romney DM. Parents' differential socialization of boys and girls: a meta-analysis. *Psychol Bull*. 1991;109:267–296.

27. Raag T, Rackliff CL. Preschoolers' awareness of social expectations of gender: relationships to toy choice. *Sex Roles*. 1198;38:685–700.

28. Shutts K, Kenward B, Falk H, Ivegran A, Fawcett C. Early preschool environments and gender: effects of gender pedagogy in Sweden. *J Exp Child Psychol*. 2017;162:1–17.

29. Goldhill O. Parents who refuse to call their newborns "girls" or "boys" are leading the gender revolution. *Quartz at Work*. https://qz.com/work/1279876/gender-neutral-parenting-aims-to-blow-up-stereotypes-from-birth/. Published June 12, 2018.

30. Always. Our epic battle #likeagirl. https://always.com/en-us/about-us/our-epic-battle-like-a-girl. Accessed November 9, 2018.

31. Newsome J. Pope warns of "ideological colonization" in transgender teachings. *CNN.com*. https://www.cnn.com/2016/10/02/world/pope-transgender-comments/index.html. Published October 2, 2016.

32. Littman L. Rapid-onset gender dysphoria in adolescents and young adults: a study of parental reports. *PLoS One*. 2018;13(8):e0202330.

33. Wadman M. New paper ignites storm over whether teens experience "rapid onset" of transgender identity. *Science Magazine.* http://www.sciencemag.org/news/2018/08/new-paper-ignites-storm-over-whether-teens-experience-rapid-onset-transgender-identity. Published August 30, 2018.

34. Rider GN, McMorris BJ, Gower AL, Coleman E, Eisenberg ME. Health and care utilization of transgender and gender nonconforming youth: a population-based study. *Pediatrics.* 2018;141(3): e20171683.

35. van Beijsterveldt CE, Hudziak JJ, Boomsma DI. Genetic and environmental influences on cross-gender behavior and relation to behavior problems: a study of Dutch twins at ages 7 and 10 years. *Arch Sex Behav.* 2006;35(6):647–658.

36. LeVay S. *Queer Science: The Use and Abuse of Research Into Homosexuality.* Cambridge, MA: MIT Press; 1996.

37. Becerra-Culqui TA, Liu Y, Nash R, et al. Mental health of transgender and gender nonconforming youth compared with their peers. *Pediatrics.* 2018;141(5):e20173845.

38. Reisner SL, Biello KB, White Hughto JM, et al. Psychiatric diagnoses and comorbidities in a diverse, multicity cohort of young transgender women: baseline findings from project lifeskills. *JAMA Pediatrics.* 2016;170(5):481–486.

39. Lowry R, Johns MM, Gordon AR, Austin SB, Robin LE, Kann LK. Nonconforming gender expression and associated mental distress and substance use among high school students. *JAMA Pediatrics.* 2018.172(11):1020–1028.

40. Baams L. Disparities for LGBTQ and gender nonconforming adolescents. *Pediatrics.* 2018;141(5):e20173004.

41. Association AP. *Diagnostic and Statistical Manual of Mental Disorders.* 4th ed., text rev. Washington, DC: American Psychiatric Association; 2000.

42. Olson KR, Durwood L, DeMeules M, McLaughlin KA. Mental health of transgender children who are supported in their identities. *Pediatrics.* 2016;137(3):e20153223.

43. Coolidge FL, Thede LL, Young SE. The heritability of gender identity disorder in a child and adolescent twin sample. *Behav Genet.* 2002;32(4):251–257.

44. Heylens G, De Cuypere G, Zucker KJ, et al. Gender identity disorder in twins: a review of the case report literature. *J Sex Medicine.* 2012;9(3):751–757.

45. Yang F, Zhu XH, Zhang Q, et al. Genomic characteristics of gender dysphoria patients and identification of rare mutations in ryr3 gene. *Sci Rep.* 2017;7(1):8339.

46. Cohen-Kettenis PT, Pfafflin F. *Transgenderism and Intersexuality in Childhood and Adolescence: Making Choices.* London, UK: SAGE; 2003.

47. de Vries AL, McGuire JK, Steensma TD, Wagenaar EC, Doreleijers TA, Cohen-Kettenis PT. Young adult psychological outcome after puberty suppression and gender reassignment. *Pediatrics.* 2014;134(4):696–704.

# Chapter 8

1. Schwarzenberg SJ, Georgieff MK. Advocacy for improving nutrition in the first 1000 days to support childhood development and adult health. *Pediatrics.* 2017;141(2):e20173716.

2. Pollitt E, Gorman KS, Engle PL, Rivera JA, Martorell R. Nutrition in early life and the fulfillment of intellectual potential. *J Nutrition.* 1995;125(4 Suppl):1111S–1118S.

3. Skinner AC, Ravanbakht SN, Skelton JA, Perrin EM, Armstrong SC. Prevalence of obesity and severe obesity in us children, 1999–2016. *Pediatrics.* 2018;143(3):pii: e20181916.

4. Ogden CL, Carroll MD, Lawman HG, et al. Trends in obesity prevalence among children and adolescents in the United States, 1988–1994 through 2013–2014. *JAMA*. 2016;315(21):2292–2299.

5. Swinburn BA, Sacks G, Hall KD, et al. The global obesity pandemic: shaped by global drivers and local environments. *Lancet*. 2011;378(9793):804–814.

6. Wardle J. Parental influences on children's diets. *Proceed Nut Society*. 1995;54(3):747–758.

7. Taylor CM, Wernimont SM, Northstone K, Emmett PM. Picky/fussy eating in children: review of definitions, assessment, prevalence and dietary intakes. *Appetite*. 2015;95:349–359.

8. Dovey TM, Staples PA, Gibson EL, Halford JC. Food neophobia and "picky/fussy" eating in children: a review. *Appetite*. 2008;50(2-3):181–193.

9. Mascola AJ, Bryson SW, Agras WS. Picky eating during childhood: a longitudinal study to age 11 years. *Eat Behaviors*. 2010;11:253–257.

10. Tharner A, Jansen PW, Kiefte-de Jong JC, et al. Toward an operative diagnosis of fussy/picky eating: a latent profile approach in a population-based cohort. *Int J Behav Nut Phys Activity*. 2014;11:14.

11. Cardona Cano S, Tiemeier H, Van Hoeken D, et al. Trajectories of picky eating during childhood: a general population study. *Int J Eat Disord*. 2015;48(6):570–579.

12. Orun E, Erdil Z, Cetinkaya T, Tufan N, Yalcin SS. Problematic eating behaviour in Turkish children aged 12–72 months: characteristics of mothers and children. *Central Eur J Pub Health*. 2012;20:257–261.

13. Xue Y, Zhao A, Cai L, et al. Growth and development in Chinese pre-schoolers with picky eating behaviour: a cross-sectional study. *PLoS One*. 2015;10(4):e0123664.

14. Carruth BR, Ziegler PJ, Gordon A, Barr SI. Prevalence of picky eaters among infants and toddlers and their caregivers' decisions about offering a new food. *J Am Diet Association*. 2004;104(1 Suppl 1):s57–s64.

15. Jansen PW, Roza SJ, Jaddoe VW, et al. Children's eating behavior, feeding practices of parents and weight problems in early childhood: results from the population-based Generation R study. *Int J Behav Nut Phys Activity*. 2012;9:130.

16. Ekstein S, Laniado D, Glick B. Does picky eating affect weight-for-length measurements in young children? *Clin Pediatrics*. 2010;49(3):217–220.

17. American Psychiatric Association. *Diagnostic and Statistical Manual of Mental Disorders*. 5th ed. Arlington, VA: American Psychiatric Publishing; 2013.

18. Le Billon K. *French Kids Eat Everything: How Our Family Moved to France, Cured Picky Eating, Banned Snacking, and Discovered 10 Simple Rules for Raising Happy Healthy Eater*. New York, NY: William Morrow; 2012.

19. Satter E. *Secrets of Feeding a Healthy Family: How to Eat, How to Raise Good Eaters, How to Cook*. 2nd ed. Madison, WI: Kelcy Press; 2008.

20. Satter E. Eating competence: definition and evidence for the Satter eating competence model. *J Nutr Educ Behav*. 2007;39(5 Suppl):S142–S153.

21. Satter E. The Ellyn Satter Institute. https://www.ellynsatterinstitute.org/. Accessed May 18, 2018.

22. Stang J, Loth KA. Parenting style and child feeding practices: potential mitigating factors in the etiology of childhood obesity. *J Am Diet Assoc*. 2011;111(9):1301–1305.

23. Rose D. *It's Not About the Broccoli: Three Habits to Teach Your Kids for a Lifetime of Healthy Eating*. New York, NY: Perigee; 2014.

24. Gidding SS, Dennison BA, Birch LL, et al. Dietary recommendations for children and adolescents: a guide for practitioners. *Pediatrics*. 2006;117(2):544–559.

25. American Academy of Pediatrics. 10 tips for parents of picky eaters. https://www. healthychildren.org/English/ages-stages/toddler/nutrition/Pages/Picky-Eaters.aspx. Accessed April 30, 2018.

26. Muth ND, Sampson S. *The Picky Eater Project: 6 Weeks to Happier, Healthier Family Mealtimes*. Elk Grove Village, IL: American Academy of Pediatrics; 2017.

27. Benjamin Neelon SE, Briley ME. Position of the American Dietetic Association: benchmarks for nutrition in child care. *J Am Diet Assoc*. 2011;111(4):607–615.

28. Eneli IU, Tylka TL, Hummel J, et al. Rationale and design of the feeding dynamic intervention (FDI) study for self-regulation of energy intake in preschoolers. *Contemp Clin Trials*. 2015;41:325–334.

29. Dowd M. "I'm president," so no more broccoli. *New York Times*. https://www.nytimes.com/ 1990/03/23/us/i-m-president-so-no-more-broccoli.html. Published March 23, 1990.

30. DeCosta P, Moller P, Frost MB, Olsen A. Changing children's eating behaviour: a review of experimental research. *Appetite*. 2017;113:327–357.

31. Galloway AT, Fiorito LM, Francis LA, Birch LL. "Finish your soup": counterproductive effects of pressuring children to eat on intake and affect. *Appetite*. 2006;46(3):318–323.

32. Hendy HM. Comparison of five teacher actions to encourage children's new food acceptance. *Ann Behav Med*. 1999;21(1):20–26.

33. Wansink B, Just DR, Payne CR, Klinger MZ. Attractive names sustain increased vegetable intake in schools. *Prev Med*. 2012;55(4):330–332.

34. Coulthard H, Sealy A. Play with your food! Sensory play is associated with tasting of fruits and vegetables in preschool children. *Appetite*. 2017;113:84–90.

35. Wilson B. *First Bite: How We Learn to Eat*. New York, NY: Basic Books; 2015.

36. Cole NC, Wang AA, Donovan SM, Lee SY, Teran-Garcia M, Team SK. Variants in chemosensory genes are associated with picky eating behavior in preschool-age children. *J Nutrigen Nutrigenomics*. 2017;10(3-4):84–92.

37. Bandini LG, Anderson SE, Curtin C, et al. Food selectivity in children with autism spectrum disorders and typically developing children. *J Pediatrics*. 2010;157(2):259–264.

38. Zucker N, Copeland W, Franz L, et al. Psychological and psychosocial impairment in preschoolers with selective eating. *Pediatrics*. 2015;136(3):e582–590.

39. Sharp WG, Burrell TL, Jaquess DL. The autism meal plan: a parent-training curriculum to manage eating aversions and low intake among children with autism. *Autism: Int J Res Pract*. 2014;18(6):712–722.

40. Johnson CR, Foldes E, DeMand A, Brooks MM. Behavioral parent training to address feeding problems in children with autism spectrum disorder: a pilot trial. *J Dev Phys Disabilit*. 2015;27(5):591–607.

41. Kuschner ES, Morton HE, Maddox BB, de Marchena A, Anthony LG, Reaven J. The buffet program: development of a cognitive behavioral treatment for selective eating in youth with autism spectrum disorder. *Clin Child Fam Psychol Rev*. 2017;20(4):403–421.

42. Constantino JN, Todd RD. Autistic traits in the general population: a twin study. *Arch Gen Psychiatry*. 2003;60(5):524–530.

43. Stafford LD, Tsang I, Lopez B, Severini M, Iacomini S. Autistic traits associated with food neophobia but not olfactory sensitivity. *Appetite*. 2017;116:584–588.

44. Rettew DC. *Child Temperament: New Thinking About the Boundary Between Traits and Illness*. New York: W. W. Norton; 2013.

45. Frank RA, van der Klaauw NJ. The contribution of chemosensory factors to individual differences in reported food preferences. *Appetite*. 1994;22(2):101–123.
46. Pliner P, Hobden K. Development of a scale to measure the trait of food neophobia in humans. *Appetite*. 1992;19(2):105–120.

# Chapter 9

1. Lansford JE. Parental divorce and children's adjustment. *Psychol Science*. 2009;4(2):140–152.
2. Miller CC. The divorce surge is over, but the myth lives on. *New York Times*. https://www.nytimes.com/2014/12/02/upshot/the-divorce-surge-is-over-but-the-myth-lives-on.html. Published December 2, 2014.
3. National Center for Family & Marriage Research. Divorce rate in the U.S.: geographic variation. https://www.bgsu.edu/content/dam/BGSU/college-of-arts-and-sciences/NCFMR/documents/FP/anderson-divorce-rate-us-geo-2016-fp-16-21.pdf. Published 2016.
4. Arkowitz H, Lilienfeld SO. Is divorce bad for children? The breakup may be painful, but most kids adjust well over time. *Sci American*. https://www.scientificamerican.com/article/is-divorce-bad-for-children/. Published March 1, 2013.
5. Wallerstein JS, Lewis JM, Blakeslee S. *The Unexpected Legacy of Divorce: A 25 Year Landmark Study*. New York, NY: Hyperion; 2000.
6. Waite LJ, Gallagher M. *The Case for Marraige: Why Married People Are Happier, Healthier, and Better Off Financially*. New York, NY: Doubleday; 2000.
7. DePaulo B. *Singled Out: How Singles Are Stereotyped, Stigmatized, and Ignored, and Still Live Happily Ever After*. New York, NY: St Martin's Press; 2006.
8. Amato PR. Reconciling divergent perspectives: Judith Wallerstein, quantitative family research, and children of divorce. *Fam Relations*. 2003;52:332–339.
9. Brown DW, Anda RF, Tiemeier H, et al. Adverse childhood experiences and the risk of premature mortality. *Am J Prev Med*. 2009;37(5):389–396.
10. Felitti VJ, Anda RF, Nordenberg D, et al. Relationship of childhood abuse and household dysfunction to many of the leading causes of death in adults: the adverse childhood experiences (ACE) study. *Am J Prev Med*. 1998;14(4):245–258.
11. Hetherington EM, Kelly J. *For Better or for Worse: Divorce Reconsidered*. New York, NY: W. W. Norton; 2002.
12. Steele F, Sigle-Rushton W, Kravdal Ø. Consequences of family disruption on children's educational outcomes in Norway. *Demography*. 2009;46(3):553–574.
13. Cherlin AJ, Chalse-Lansdale PL, McCrae C. Effects of parental divorce on mental health throughout the life course. *Am Sociol Rev*. 1998;63:239–249.
14. Amato PR, Anthony CJ. Estimating the effects of parental divorce and death with fixed effects models. *J Marriage Family*. 2014;76(2):370–386.
15. Kelly JB. Children's adjustment in conflicted marriage and divorce: a decade review of research. *J Am Acad Child Adolesc Psychiatry*. 2000;39(8):963–973.
16. Amato PR. Children of divorce in the 1990s: an update of the Amato and Keith (1991) meta-analysis. *J Fam Psychology*. 2001;15:355–370.
17. Wallerstein JS, Blakeslee S. *Second Chances: Men, Women, and Children a Decade After Divorce*. Boston, MA: Houghton Mifflin; 1989.
18. Jocklin V, McGue M, Lykken DT. Personality and divorce: a genetic analysis. *J Pers Soc Psychol*. 1996;71(2):288–299.

19. O.Connor TG, Caspi A, DeFries JC, Plomin R. Are associations between parental divorce and children's adjustment genetically mediated? An adoption study. *Dev Psychol.* 2000;36:429–437.

20. D'Onofrio BM, Turkheimer E, Emery RE, Maes HH, Silberg J, Eaves LJ. A children of twins study of parental divorce and offspring psychopathology. *J Child Psychol Psychiatry.* 2007;48(7):667–675.

21. Hetherington EM. Divorce and the adjustment of children. *Pediat Rev.* 2005;26(5):163–169.

22. Lansford JE, Malone PS, Castellino DR, Dodge KA, Pettit GS, Bates JE. Trajectories of internalizing, externalizing, and grades for children who have and have not experienced their parents' divorce. *J Fam Psychology.* 2006;20:292–301.

23. Malone PS, Lansford JE, Castellino DR, et al. Divorce and child behavior problems: applying latent change score models to life event data. *Struct Equation Model.* 2004;11(3):401–423.

24. Hetherington EM, Bridges M, Insabella GM. What matters? What does not? Five perspectives on the association between marital transitions and children's adjustment. *Am Psychol.* 1998;53(2):167–184.

25. Allison PD, Furstenberg FF, Jr. How marital dissolution affects children: variations by age and sex. *Dev Psychology.* 1989;25:540–549.

26. Amato PR, Cheadle J. The long reach of divorce: divorce and child well-being across three generations. *J Marriage Family.* 2005;67:191–206.

27. Amato PR, Keith B. Parental divorce and the well-being of children: a meta-analysis. *Psychol Bull.* 1991;110:26–46.

28. Chase-Lansdale L, Cherlin AJ, Kiernan KE. The long-term effects of parental divorce on the mental health of young adults: a developmental perspective. *Child Dev.* 1995;66:1614–1634.

29. Cherlin AJ, Furstenberg FF, Jr., Chase-Lansdale L, et al. Longitudinal studies of effects of divorce on children in Great Britain and the United States. *Science.* 1991;252(5011):1386–1389.

30. Kasen S, Cohen P, Brook JS, Hartmark C. A multiple-risk interaction model: effects of temperament and divorce on psychiatric disorders in children. *J Abnorm Child Psychol.* 1996;24(2):121–150.

31. Lengua LJ, Wolchik SA, Sandles IN, West SG. The additive and interactive effects of parenting and temperament in predicting adjustment problems of children of divorce. *J Clin Child Psychology.* 2000;29:232–244.

32. Buchanan CM, Maccoby EE, Dornbusch SM. *Adolescents After Divorce.* Cambridge, MA: Harvard University Press; 1996.

33. Videon TM. The effects of parent–adolescent relationships and parental separation on adolescent well-being. *J Marriage Fam.* 2002;64:489–503.

34. Hetherington EM, Stanley-Hagan M. The adjustment of children with divorced parents: a risk and resiliency perspective. *J Child Psychol Psychiatry.* 1999;40(1):129–140.

35. Amato PR, Booth A. A prospective study of divorce and parent–child relationships. *J Marriage Family.* 1996;58:356–365.

36. Amato PR, Gilbreth JG. Nonresident fathers and children's well-being: a meta-analysis. *J Marriage Family.* 1999;61(3):557–573.

37. Martinez CRJ, Forgatch MS. Adjusting to change: linking family structure transitions with parenting and boys' adjustment. *J Family Psychology.* 2002;16:107–117.

38. Booth A, Amato PR. Parental predivorce relations and offspring postdivorce well-being. *J Marriage Fam.* 2001;63:197–212.

39. Vandewater EA, Lansford JE. Influences of family structure and parental conflict on children's well-being. *Fam Relations.* 1998;47:323–330.

40. Moroni G. *Explaining Divorce Gaps in Cognitive and Non-Cognitive Skills of Children.* Paper presented at the Royal Economic Society Conference in Bristol, UK, April, 2017.

41. Amato PR, Loomis LS, Booth A. Parental divorce, marital conflict, and offspring well-being during early adulthood. *Soc Forces.* 1995;73:895–915.

42. Bauserman R. Child adjustment in joint-custody versus sole custody arrangements: a meta-analytic review. *J Fam Psychology.* 2002;16:91–102.

43. Li J-CA. *The Kids Are OK: Divorce and Children's Behavior Problems.* Santa Monica, CA: Rand Corporation;2007.

# Chapter 10

1. Global Initiative to End all Corporeal Punishment of Children. Global progress towards prohibiting all corporal punishment. https://endcorporalpunishment.org/. Published January, 2018.

2. Elgar FJ, Donnelly PD, Michaelson V, et al. Corporal punishment bans and physical fighting in adolescents: an ecological study of 88 countries. *BMJ Open.* 2018;8(9):e021616.

3. Gershoff ET, Font SA. Corporal punishment in U.S. Public schools: prevalence, disparities in use, and status in state and federal policy. *Soc Policy Rep.* 2016;30(1):1–25.

4. Straus MA, Mather AK. Social change and change in approval of corporal punishment by parents from 1968 to 1994. In: Frehsee D, Horn W, Bussman KD, eds. *Family Violence Against Children: A Challenge for Society.* New York, NY: deGruyter; 1996: 91–105.

5. Cuddy E, Reeves RV. Hitting kids: American parenting and physical punishment. *Brookings Institution.* https://www.brookings.edu/research/hitting-kids-american-parenting-and-physical-punishment/. Published November 6, 2014.

6. Smith TW, Davern M, Freese J. Morgan SL. The general social survey. *NORC at the University of Chicago.* http://gss.norc.org/. Accessed February 11, 2018.

7. Clement S. Millennials like to spank their kids just as much as their parents did. *Washington Post.* https://www.washingtonpost.com/news/wonk/wp/2015/03/05/millennials-like-to-spank-their-kids-just-as-much-as-their-parents-did/. Published March 5, 2015.

8. Schenck ER, Lyman RD, Bodin SD. Ethical beliefs, attitudes, and professional practices of psychologists regarding parental use of corporal punishment: a survey. *Child Serv.* 2000;3:23–38.

9. healthychildren.org. What's the best way to discipline my child? https://www.healthychildren.org/English/family-life/family-dynamics/communication-discipline/Pages/Disciplining-Your-Child.aspx. Accessed Dec 3, 2020.

10. Sege RD, Siegel BS, et al. Effective discipline to raise healthy children. *Pediatrics.* 2018;142(6):e20183112.

11. American Academy of Child & Adolescent Psychiatry. Corporeal punishment. https://www.aacap.org/aacap/Policy_Statements/2012/Policy_Statement_on_Corporal_Punishment.aspx. Published 2012.

12. American Psychological Association. Resolution on physical discipline of children by parents. https://www.apa.org/about/policy/physical-discipline.pdf. Accessed February 24, 2020.

13. American College of Pediatricians. Corporal punishment: a scientific review of its use in discipline. http://www.acpeds.org/the-college-speaks/position-statements/parenting-issues/corporal-punishment-a-scientific-review-of-its-use-in-discipline. Accessed December 3, 2020.

14. Afifi TO, Ford D, Gershoff ET, et al. Spanking and adult mental health impairment: the case for the designation of spanking as an adverse childhood experience. *Child Abuse Neglect*. 2017;71:24–31.

15. Gershoff ET, Grogan-Kaylor A. Spanking and child outcomes: old controversies and new meta-analyses. *J Fam Psychol*. 2016;30(4):453–469.

16. Paolucci EO, Violato C. A meta-analysis of the published research on the affective, cognitive, and behavioral effects of corporal punishment. *J Psychology*. 2004;138:197–221.

17. Gershoff ET. Corporal punishment by parents and associated child behaviors and experiences: a meta-analytic and theoretical review. *Psychol Bull*. 2002;128:539–579.

18. Ferguson CJ. Spanking, corporal punishment and negative longterm outcomes: a meta-analytic review of longitudinal studies. *Clin Psychol Rev*. 2013;33:196–208.

19. Larzelere RE, Kuhn BR. Comparing child outcomes of physical punishment and alternative disciplinary tactics: a meta-analysis. *Clin Child Fam Psychol Rev*. 2005;8:1–37.

20. Press A. A new look at the effects of spanking. *New York Times*. http://www.nytimes.com/2002/07/09/health/a-new-look-at-effects-of-spanking.html. Published July 9, 2002.

21. Vries L. Spanking may cause long-term harm. *CBS News*. https://www.cbsnews.com/news/spanking-may-cause-long-term-harm/. Published June 26, 2002.

22. Baumrind D, Larzelere RE, Cowan PA. Ordinary physical punishment: is it harmful? Comment on Gershoff (2002). *Psychol Bull*. 2002;128(4):580–589.

23. Beauchaine TP, Webster-Stratton C, Reid MJ. Mediators, moderators, and predictors of 1-year outcomes among children treated for early-onset conduct problems: a latent growth curve analysis. *J Consult Clin Psychol*. 2005;73(3):371–388.

24. Larzelere RE, Kuhn BR, Johnson B. The intervention selection bias: an underrecognized confound in intervention research. *Psychol Bull*. 2004;130(2):289–303.

25. American College of Pediatricians. *Spanking: a valid option for parents*. https://acpeds.org/assets/imported/Spanking-Press-release-for-website.pdf. Accessed December 3, 2020.

26. Roberts MW, Powers SW. Adjusting chair timeout enforcement procedures for oppositional children *Behav Therapy*. 1990;21:257–271.

27. Day DE, Robers MW. An analysis of the physical punishment component of a parent training program. *J Abnorm Child Psychology*. 1983;11(1):141–152.

28. Gershoff ET, Grogan-Kaylor A, Lansford JE, et al. Parent discipline practices in an international sample: associations with child behaviors and moderation by perceived normativeness. *Child Dev*. 2010;81(2):487–502.

29. Temple JR, Choi HJ, Reuter T, et al. Childhood corporal punishment and future perpetration of physical dating violence. *Journal Pediatrics*. 2018;194:233–237.

30. Gershoff ET, Goodman GS, Miller-Perrin CL, Holden GW, Jackson Y, Kazdin AE. The strength of the causal evidence against physical punishment of children

and its implications for parents, psychologists, and policymakers. *Am Psychol.* 2018;73(5):626–638.

31. Finkelhor D, Turner HA, Shattuck A, Hamby SL. Prevalence of childhood exposure to violence, crime, and abuse: results from the national survey of children's exposure to violence. *JAMA Pediatrics.* 2015;169(8):746–754.

32. Twenge JM. Have smartphones destroyed a generation? *The Atlantic.* https://www.theatlantic.com/magazine/archive/2017/09/has-the-smartphone-destroyed-a-generation/534198/. Published September 2017.

33. Trumbull DA. Discipline of the child series: disciplinary spanking. https://acpeds.org/assets/imported/Disciplinary-Spanking1.pdf. Published 2006.

34. Smith JR, Brooks-Gunn J. Correlates and consequences of harsh discipline for young children. *Arch Pediatr Adolesc Med.* 1997;151(8):777–786.

35. Deater-Deckard K, Dodge KA, Bates JE, Pettit GS. Physical discipline among African American and European American mothers: links to children's externalizing behaviors. *Devel Psychology.* 1996;32(6):1065–1072.

36. Gunnoe ML, Mariner CL. Toward a developmental-contextual model of the effects of parental spanking on children's aggression. *Arch Pediatr Adolesc Med.* 1997;151(8):768–775.

37. Stacks AM, Oshio T, Gerard J, Roe J. The moderating effect of parental warmth on the association between spanking and child aggression: a longitudinal approach. *Infant Child Dev.* 2009;18:189–194.

38. Lansford JE, Deater-Deckard K, Dodge KA, Bates JE, Pettit GS. Ethnic differences in the link between physical discipline and later adolescent externalizing behaviors. *J Child Psychol Psychiatry.* 2004;45(4):801–812.

39. McLoyd VC, Smith J. Physical discipline and behavior problems in African American, European American, and Hispanic children: emotional support as a moderator. *J Marriage Family.* 2002;64(1):40–53.

40. Grogan-Kaylor A. Corporal punishment and the growth trajectory of children's anti-social behavior. *Child Maltreat.* 2005;10(3):283–292.

41. Okuzono S, Fujiwara T, Kato T, Kawachi I. Spanking and subsequent behavioral problems in toddlers: a propensity score-matched, prospective study in Japan. *Child Abuse Neglect.* 2017;69:62–71.

42. Rohner RP, Kean KJ, Cournoyer DE. Effects of corporal punishment, perceived care-taker warmth, and cultural beliefs on the psychological adjustment of children in St. Kitts, West Indies. *J Marriage Family.* 1991;53:681–693.

43. Ripoll-Nunez KJ, Rohner RP. Corporal punishment in cross-cultural perspective: directions for a research agenda. *Cross Cult Research.* 2006;40(3):220–249.

44. Mendez M, Durtschi J, Neppl TK, Stith SM. Corporal punishment and externalizing behaviors in toddlers: the moderating role of positive and harsh parenting. *J Fam Psychol.* 2016;30(8):887–895.

45. Barnes JC, Boutwell BB, Beaver KM, Gibson CL. Analyzing the origins of childhood externalizing behavioral problems. *Dev Psychol.* 2013;49(12):2272–2284.

46. Rutter M, Moffitt TE, Caspi A. Gene-environment interplay and psychopathology: multiple varieties but real effects. *J Child Psychol Psychiatry.* 2006;47(3-4):226–261.

47. Klahr AM, Burt SA. Elucidating the etiology of individual differences in parenting: a meta-analysis of behavioral genetic research. *Psychol Bull.* 2014;140(2):544–586.

48. Xu Y, Farver JA, Zhang Z. Temperament, harsh and indulgent parenting, and Chinese children's proactive and reactive aggression. *Child Dev.* 2009;80(1):244–258.

49. Colder CR, Lochman JE, Wells KC. The moderating effects of children's fear and activity level on relations between parenting practices and childhood symptomatology. *J Abnorm Child Psychol.* 1997;25(3):251–263.

50. Gardner F, Leijten P. Incredible years parenting interventions: current effectiveness research and future directions. *Curr Opin Psychol.* 2017;15:99–104.

51. McMahon RJ, Forehand RL. *Helping the Noncompliant Child: Family Based Treatment for Oppositional Behavior.* New York, NY: Guilford Press; 2003.

52. Siegel DJ, Bryson TP. "Time-outs" are hurting your child. *Time Magazine.* http://time.com/3404701/discipline-time-out-is-not-good/. Published September 23, 2014.

53. Siegel DJ, Bryson TP. *No Drama Discipine: A Whole-Brain Way to Calm the Chaos and Nurture Your Child's Developing Mind.* New York, NY: Bantam Books; 2014.

54. Siegel D. You said what about time-outs?! *Dr. Dan Siegel.* http://www.drdansiegel.com/blog/2014/10/29/you-said-what-about-time-outs/. Published October 29, 2014.

55. Allen DG. Time is up for timeouts. *CNN.com.* https://www.cnn.com/2018/02/16/health/time-out-parenting-go-ask-your-dad/index.html. Published February 16, 2018.

56. Bates JE, Pettit GS, Dodge KA, Ridge B. Interaction of temperamental resistance to control and restrictive parenting in the development of externalizing behavior. *Dev Psychology.* 1998;34:982–995.

57. Greene RW. *The Explosive Child: A New Approach for Understanding and Parenting Easily Frustrated, "Chronically Inflexible" Children.* New York, NY: Harper Collins; 1998.

# Chapter 11

1. Twenge JM. Have smartphones destroyed a generation? *The Atlantic.* https://www.theatlantic.com/magazine/archive/2017/09/has-the-smartphone-destroyed-a-generation/534198/. Published September 2017.

2. Cooper A. Groundbreaking study examines effects of screen time on kids. *60 Minutes.* https://www.cbsnews.com/news/groundbreaking-study-examines-effects-of-screen-time-on-kids-60-minutes/. Published December 9, 2018.

3. Radesky JS, Eisenberg S, Kistin CJ, et al. Overstimulated consumers or next-generation learners? Parent tensions about child mobile technology use. *Ann Fam Med.* 2016;14(6):503–508.

4. American Academy of Pediatrics, Council on Communication and Media. Media and young minds. *Pediatrics.* 2016;138(5): e20162591.

5. Christakis DA. Interactive media use at younger than the age of 2 years: time to rethink the American Academy of Pediatrics guideline? *JAMA Pediatrics.* 2014;168(5):399–400.

6. Ferguson C. New American Academy of Pediatrics screen time recommendations still don't make a passing grade. *Huffington Post.* https://www.huffpost.com/entry/new-american-academy-of-pediatrics-screen-time-recommendations_b_5814a3fae4b08301d33e0a16. Published October 31, 2016.

7. Common Sense Media. Children, teens, and reading: a common sense media brief. https://www.commonsensemedia.org/research/children-teens-and-reading. Published May 12, 2014.

8. Olson CK, Kutner L, Beresin E. Children and video games: how much do we know? *Psychiatric Times.* http://www.psychiatrictimes.com/child-adolescent-psychiatry/children-and-video-games-how-much-do-we-know/page/0/2. Published October 1, 2007.

9. Bandura A, Ross D, Ross SA. Transmission of aggression through imitation of aggressive models. *J Abnorm Soc Psychology.* 1961;63:575–582.

10. Dillon KP, Bushman BJ. Effects of exposure to gun violence in movies on children's interest in real guns. *JAMA Pediatrics.* 2017;171(11):1057–1062.

11. Christakis DA, Garrison MM, Herrenkohl T, et al. Modifying media content for preschool children: a randomized controlled trial. *Pediatrics.* 2013;131(3):431–438.

12. Zimmerman FJ, Christakis DA. Children's television viewing and cognitive outcomes: a longitudinal analysis of national data. *Arch Pediatr Adolesc Med.* 2005;159(7):619–625.

13. Pagani LS, Fitzpatrick C, Barnett TA, Dubow E. Prospective associations between early childhood television exposure and academic, psychosocial, and physical well-being by middle childhood. *Arch Pediatr Adolesc Med.* 2010;164(5):425–431.

14. Smith S, Ferguson CJ. The effects of violent media on children. In: Beresin EV, Olson CK, eds. *Child and Adolescent Psychiatry and the Media.* St. Louis, MO: Elsevier; 2019: 1–9.

15. Stiglic N, Viner RM. Effects of screentime on the health and well-being of children and adolescents: a systematic review of reviews. *BMJ Open.* 2019;9(1):e023191.

16. Unsworth G, Devilly GJ, Ward T. The effect of playing violent video games on adolescents: should parents be quaking in their boots? *Psychol Crime Law.* 2007;13(4):383–394.

17. Anderson CA, Shibuya A, Ihori N, et al. Violent video game effects on aggression, empathy, and prosocial behavior in eastern and western countries: a meta-analytic review. *Psychol Bull.* 2010;136(2):151–173.

18. Hilgard J, Engelhart CR, Rouder JN. Overstated evidence for short-term effects of violent games on affect and behavior: a reanalysis of Anderson et al. (2010). *Psychol Bull.* 2017;143(7):757–774.

19. Strasburger VC, Jordan AB, Donnerstein E. Children, adolescents, and the media: health effects. *Ped Clin North America.* 2012;59(3):533–587.

20. American Academy of Pediatrics, Council on Communication and Media. From the American Academy of Pediatrics: policy statement—media and violence. *Pediatrics.* 2009;124(5):1495–1503.

21. Christakis DA, Zimmerman FJ, DiGiuseppe DL, McCarty CA. Early television exposure and subsequent attentional problems in children. *Pediatrics.* 2004;113(4):708–713.

22. Ra CK, Cho J, Stone MD, et al. Association of digital media use with subsequent symptoms of attention-deficit/hyperactivity disorder among adolescents. *JAMA.* 2018;320(3):255–263.

23. Suchert V, Hanewinkel R, Isensee B. Sedentary behavior and indicators of mental health in school-aged children and adolescents: a systematic review. *Prev Med.* 2015;76:48–57.

24. Nikkelen SW, Valkenburg PM, Huizinga M, Bushman BJ. Media use and ADHD-related behaviors in children and adolescents: a meta-analysis. *Dev Psychol.* 2014;50(9):2228–2241.

25. Johnson JG, Cohen P, Kasen S, Brook JS. Extensive television viewing and the development of attention and learning difficulties during adolescence. *Arch Pediatr Adolesc Med.* 2007;161(5):480–486.

26. Swing EL, Gentile DA, Anderson CA, Walsh DA. Television and video game exposure and the development of attention problems. *Pediatrics.* 2010;126(2):214–221.

27. Madigan S, Browne D, Racine N, Mori C, Tough S. Association between screen time and children's performance on a developmental screening test. *JAMA Pediatrics.* 2019;173(3):244–250.

28. Hutton JS, Dudley J, Horowitz-Kraus T, et al. Associations between screen-based media use and brain white matter integrity in preschool-aged children. *JAMA Pediatrics.* 2019;174(1):e193869.

29. Walsh JJ, Barnes JD, Cameron JD, et al. Associations between 24 hour movement behaviours and global cognition in us children: a cross-sectional observational study. *Lancet Child Adolesc Health.* 2018;2(11):783–791.

30. Mishra J, Sagar R, Joseph AA, Gazzaley A, Merzenich MM. Training sensory signal-to-noise resolution in children with ADHD in a global mental health setting. *Transl Psychiatry.* 2016;6(4):e781.

31. Christakis DA, Ramirez JS, Ramirez JM. Overstimulation of newborn mice leads to behavioral differences and deficits in cognitive performance. *Sci Rep.* 2012;2:546.

32. Hamilton J. Heavy screen time rewires young brains, for better and worse. NPR. https://www.npr.org/sections/health-shots/2016/11/19/502610055/heavy-screen-time-rewires-young-brains-for-better-and-worse. Published November 19, 2016.

33. Kearney MS, Levine PB. Early childhood education by MOOC: lessons from Sesame Street. *National Bureau of Economic Research.* http://www.nber.org/papers/w21229.pdf. Published June, 2015.

34. Wright JC, Huston AC, Scantlin R, Kotler J. The early window project: Sesame Street prepares children for school. In: Fisch S, Truglio R, eds. *"G" Is for Growing: Thirty Years of Research on Children and Sesame Street.* Mahwah, NJ: Erlbaum; 2009: 97–114.

35. Ferguson CJ. The good, the bad and the ugly: a meta-analytic review of positive and negative effects of violent video games. *Psychiatr Q.* 2007;78(4):309–316.

36. Dye MW, Green CS, Bavelier D. Increasing speed of processing with action video games. *Curr Dir Psychol Sci.* 2009;18(6):321–326.

37. Kuhn S, Gleich T, Lorenz RC, Lindenberger U, Gallinat J. Playing Super Mario induces structural brain plasticity: gray matter changes resulting from training with a commercial video game. *Mol Psychiatry.* 2014;19(2):265–271.

38. Kuhn S, Lorenz R, Banaschewski T, et al. Positive association of video game playing with left frontal cortical thickness in adolescents. *PLoS One.* 2014;9(3):e91506.

39. Wartella EA, Lauricella AR. Should babies be watching television and DVDs? *Pediatric Clin N Am.* 2012;59(3):613–621, vii.

40. Richert RA, Robb MB, Fender JG, Wartella E. Word learning from baby videos. *Arch Pediatr Adolesc Med.* 2010;164(5):432–437.

41. Zimmerman FJ, Christakis DA, Meltzoff AN. Associations between media viewing and language development in children under age 2 years. *J Pediatrics.* 2007;151(4):364–368.

42. DeLoache JS, Chiong C, Sherman K, et al. Do babies learn from baby media? *Psychol Sci.* 2010;21(11):1570–1574.

43. Reid Chassiakos YL, Radesky J, Christakis D, et al. Children and adolescents and digital media. *Pediatrics*. 2016;138(5).

44. Mendelsohn AL, Brockmeyer CA, Dreyer BP, Fierman AH, Berkule-Silberman SB, Tomopoulos S. Do verbal interactions with infants during electronic media exposure mitigate adverse impacts on their language development as toddlers? *Infant Child Dev*. 2010;19(6):577–593.

45. Gil-Rivas V, Silver RC, Holman EA, McIntosh DN, Poulin M. Parental response and adolescent adjustment to the September 11, 2001 terrorist attacks. *J Traum Stress*. 2007;20(6):1063–1068.

46. van der Molen JH, Bushman BJ. Children's direct fright and worry reactions to violence in fiction and news television programs. *J Pediatrics*. 2008;153(3):420–424.

47. Otto MW, Henin A, Hirshfeld-Becker DR, Pollack MH, Biederman J, Rosenbaum JF. Posttraumatic stress disorder symptoms following media exposure to tragic events: impact of 9/11 on children at risk for anxiety disorders. *J Anxiety Disord*. 2007;21(7):888–902.

48. Sugawara M, Matsumoto S, Murohashi H, Sakai A, Isshiki N. Trajectories of early television contact in japan: relationship with preschoolers' externalizing problems. *J Childr Media*. 2015;9(4):453–471.

49. Chen B, Bernard JY, Padmapriya N, et al. Associations between early-life screen viewing and 24 hour movement behaviours: findings from a longitudinal birth cohort study. *Lancet Child Adolesc Health*. 2020;4(3):201–209.

50. Przybylski AK, Rigby CS, Ryan RM. A motivational model for video game engagement. *Rev Gen Psychology*. 2010;14(2):154–166.

51. APA Task Force on Violent Media. Technical report on the review of the violent video game literature. http://www.apa.org/pi/families/violent-media.aspx. Published August 2015.

52. Hudziak JJ, Rudiger LP, Neale MC, Heath AC, Todd RD. A twin study of inattentive, aggressive, and anxious/depressed behaviors. *J Am Acad Child Adolesc Psychiatry*. 2000;39(4):469–476.

53. Hudziak JJ, van Beijsterveldt CE, Bartels M, et al. Individual differences in aggression: genetic analyses by age, gender, and informant in 3-, 7-, and 10-year-old Dutch twins. *Behav Genet*. 2003;33(5):575–589.

54. Alia-Klein N, Wang GJ, Preston-Campbell RN, et al. Reactions to media violence: it's in the brain of the beholder. *PLoS One*. 2014;9(9):e107260.

55. Markey PM, Markey CN. Vulnerability to violent video games: a review and integration of personality research. *Rev Gen Psychology*. 2010;14(2):82–91.

56. Ferguson C, Olson C. Video game violence use among "vulnerable" populations: the impact of violent games on delinquency and bullying among children with clinically elevated depression or attention deficit symptoms. *J Youth Adolescence*. 2014;43:127–136.

57. Kirsh SJ. The effects of violent video games on adolescents; the overlooked influence of development. *Aggress Viol Behavior*. 2003;8:377–389.

58. Gilissen R, Bakermans-Kranenburg MJ, van IMH, van der Veer R. Parent–child relationship, temperament, and physiological reactions to fear-inducing film clips: further evidence for differential susceptibility. *J Exp Child Psychol*. 2008;99(3):182–195.

# Chapter 12

1. Kohn A. 5 reasons to stop saying "good job!" *Young Children*. Available at https://www.alfiekohn.org/article/five-reasons-stop-saying-good-job/. Published September 2001.

2. Donnellan MB, Trzesniewski KH, Robins RW. Self-esteem: enduring issues and controversies. In: Chamorro-Premuzic SvS, Furnham A, eds. *The Wiley-Blackwell Handbook of Individual Differences*. New York, NY: Wiley-Blackwell; 2011: 718–746.

3. Branden N. *The Psychology of Self-Esteem: A Revolutionary Approach to Self-Understanding That Launched a New Era in Modern Psychology*. San Francisco, CA: Jossey-Bass; 2001.

4. Smelser NJ. Self-esteem and social problems: an introduction. In: Mecca AM, Smelser NJ, Vasconcellos J, eds. *The Social Importance of Self-Esteem*. Berkeley, CA: University of California Press; 1989: 1–23.

5. Baumeister RF, Campbell JD, Krueger JI, Vohs KD. Does high self-esteem cause better performance, interpersonal success, happiness, or healthier lifestyles? *Psychol Sci Public Interest*. 2003;4(1):1–44.

6. Donnellan MB, Trzesniewski KH, Robins RW, Moffitt TE, Caspi A. Low self-esteem is related to aggression, antisocial behavior, and delinquency. *Psychol Sci*. 2005;16(4):328–335.

7. Fergusson DM, Horwood LJ. Male and female offending trajectories. *Dev Psychopathology*. 2002;14(1):159–177.

8. Masselink M, Van Roekel E, Oldehinkel AJ. Self-esteem in early adolescence as predictor of depressive symptoms in late adolescence and early adulthood: the mediating role of motivational and social factors. *J Youth Adolesc*. 2017;45(2): 932–946.

9. Orth U, Robins RW, Meier LL, Conger RD. Refining the vulnerability model of low self-esteem and depression: disentangling the effects of genuine self-esteem and narcissism. *J Pers Soc Psychol*. 2016;110(1):133–149.

10. Orth U, Robins RW, Roberts BW. Low self-esteem prospectively predicts depression in adolescence and young adulthood. *J Pers Soc Psychol*. 2008;95(3):695–708.

11. Sowislo JF, Orth U. Does low self-esteem predict depression and anxiety? A meta-analysis of longitudinal studies. *Psychol Bull*. 2013;139(1):213–240.

12. Diener E, Diener M. Cross-cultural correlates of life satisfaction and self-esteem. *J Pers Soc Psychol*. 1995;68(4):653–663.

13. Chen SX, Cheung FM, Bond MH, Leung JW. Going beyond self-esteem to predict life satisfaction: the Chinese case. *Asia J Soc Psychology*. 2006;9(1):24–35.

14. Dweck C. Caution—praise can be dangerous. *Am Educator*. 1999;23(1):4–9.

15. Seligman MEP. *The Optimistic Child: A Proven Program to Safeguard Children Against Depression and Build Lifelong Resilience*. New York, NY: Houghton Mifflin; 1995.

16. Centers for Disease Control and Prevention. Praise, imitation, and description. https://www.cdc.gov/parents/essentials/communication/goodbehavior-praise.html. Published 2017.

17. Ginsburg KR, Jablow MM. *Building Resilience in Children and Teens: Giving Kids Roots and Wings*. 3rd ed. Elk Grove Village, IL: American Academy of Pediatrics; 2015.

18. Pruitt D. *Your Child: What Every Parent Needs to Know*. New York, NY: American Academy of Child and Adolescent Psychiatry; 1998.

19. National Research Council and Institute of Medicine. *Preventing Mental, Emotional, and Behavioral Disorders Among Young People: Progress and Possibilities*. Washington, DC: National Academies Press; 2009.

20. Jackson C, Henriksen L, Foshee VA. The authoritative parenting index: predicting health risk behaviors among children and adolescents. *Health Educ Behavior.* 1998;25(3):319–337.

21. Owen DJ, Slep AMS, Heyman RE. The effect of praise, positive nonverbal response, reprimand, and negative nonverbal response on child compliance: a systematic review. *Child Dev.* 2012;15:364–385.

22. Forehand RL, Long N. *Parenting the Strong Willed Child.* New York, NY: McGraw-Hill; 2010.

23. Thomas R, Abell B, Webb HJ, Avdagic E, Zimmer-Gembeck MJ. Parent–child interaction therapy: a meta-analysis. *Pediatrics.* 2017;140(3): e20170352.

24. Gardner F, Leijten P. Incredible years parenting interventions: current effectiveness research and future directions. *Curr Opin Psychol.* 2017;15:99–104.

25. Dweck CS. *Mindset: The New Psychology of Success.* New York, NY: Random House; 2006.

26. Giles JW, Heyman GD. Preschoolers' beliefs about the stability of antisocial behavior: implications for navigating social challenges. *Soc Development.* 2003;12:182–197.

27. Heyman GD, Dweck CS. Children's thinking about traits: implications for judgments of the self and others. *Child Dev.* 1998;69:391–403.

28. Cimpian A. The impact of generic language about ability on children's achievement motivation. *Dev Psychol.* 2007;46:1333–1340.

29. Corpus J, Leeper MR. The effects of person versus performance praise on children's motivation: gender and age as moderating factors. *Educ Psychology.* 2007;27: 487–508.

30. Zentall SR, Morris, B. "Good job, you're so smart": the effects of inconsistency of praise type on young children's motivation. *J Exp Child Psychol.* 2010;107:155–163.

31. Henderlong J, Lepper MR. The effects of praise on children's intrinsic motivation: a review and synthesis. *Psychol Bull.* 2002;128(5):774–795.

32. Kamins ML, Dweck CS. Person versus process praise and criticism: implications for contingent self-worth and coping. *Dev Psychol.* 1999;35:835–847.

33. Gunderson EA, Gripshover SJ, Romero C, Dweck CS, Goldin-Meadow S, Levine SC. Parent praise to 1- to 3-year-olds predicts children's motivational frameworks 5 years later. *Child Dev.* 2013;84(5):1526–1541.

34. Gunderson EA, Sorhagen NS, Gripshover SJ, Dweck CS, Goldin-Meadow S, Levine SC. Parent praise to toddlers predicts fourth grade academic achievement via children's incremental mindsets. *Dev Psychol.* 2017;84(5):1526–1541.

35. Skipper Y, Douglas K. Is no praise good praise? Effects of positive feedback on children's and university students' responses to subsequent failures. *Br J Educ Psychol.* 2012;82(Pt 2):327–339.

36. Mueller CM, Dweck CS. Praise for intelligence can undermine children's motivation and performance. *J Pers Soc Psychol.* 1998;75(1):33–52.

37. Grusec J, Redler E. Attribution, reinforcement, and altruism: a developmental analysis. *Dev Psychology.* 1980;16(5):525–534.

38. Bryan CJ, Master A, Walton GM. "Helping" versus "being a helper": invoking the self to increase helping in young children. *Child Dev.* 2014;85(5):1836–1842.

39. Bryan CJ, Adams GS, Benoit M. When cheating would make you a cheater: implicating the self prevents unethical behavior. *J Exper Psychology.* 2013;142(4):1001–1005.

40. Rhoades M. Will praising character help us raise moral children? *Huffington Post.* https://www.huffingtonpost.com/marjorie-rhodes-phd/will-praising-character-help-us-raise-moral-children_b_5234952.html. Published April 29, 2014.

41. Cimpian A, Arce HM, Markman EM, Dweck CS. Subtle linguistic cues affect children's motivation. *Psychol Sci.* 2007;18(4):314–316.

42. Levy SR, Dweck CS. The impact of children's static versus dynamic conceptions of people on stereotype formation. *Child Dev.* 1999;70:1163–1180.

43. Mok MMC, Kennedy KJ, Moore PJ. Academic attribution of secondary students: gender, year level and achievement level. *Educ Psychology.* 2011;31:87–104.

44. Robins RW, Donnellan MB, Widaman KF, Conger RD. Evaluating the link between self-esteem and temperament in Mexican origin early adolescents. *J Adolescence.* 2010;33(3):403–410.

45. Youngs BB. *How to Develop Self-Esteem in Your Child: Six Vital Ingredients.* New York, NY: Faucett Columbine; 1991.

46. Brummelman E, Crocker J, Bushman BJ. The praise paradox: when and why praise backfires in children with low self-esteem. *Child Dev Perspectives.* 2016;10(2):111–115.

47. Irving J. *The Cider House Rules.* New York, NY: William Morrow; 1985.

48. Farmer B. Nashville's newest charter school embraces black empowerment. http://www.kipp.org/news/nashvilles-newest-charter-school-embraces-black-empowerment/. Published November 27, 2017.

49. Barish K. Are our children overpraised? A guide to raising children with confidence and resilience. *Child Mind Institute.* https://childmind.org/article/are-our-children-overpraised/

50. Burkhouse KL, Uhrlass DJ, Stone LB, Knopik VS, Gibb BE. Expressed emotion-criticism and risk of depression onset in children. *J Clin Child Adolesc Psychol.* 2012;41(6):771–777.

51. Brennan PA, Hall J, Bor W, Najman JM, Williams G. Integrating biological and social processes in relationship to early-onset persistent aggression in boys and girls. *Dev Psychology.* 2003;39:309–323.

52. Rajyaguru P, Moran P, Cordero M, Pearson R. Disciplinary parenting practice and child mental health: evidence from the UK Millennium Cohort Study. *J Am Acad Child Adolesc Psychiatry.* 2019;58(1):108–116.

53. Zenger J, Folkman J. The ideal praise-to-criticism ratio. *Harvard Bus Rev.* https://hbr.org/2013/03/the-ideal-praise-to-criticism. Published March 25, 2013.

54. Fredrickson BL, Losada MF. Positive affect and the complex dynamics of human flourishing. *Am Psychol.* 2005;60(7):678–686.

# Chapter 13

1. Doran GT. There's a S.M.A.R.T. Way to write management's goals and objectives. *Manage Rev.* 1981;70(11):35–36.

2. Deming WE. *The New Economics.* Cambridge, MA: Massachusetts Institute of Technology Press; 1993.

3. Langley G, Nolan K, Nolan TR. The foundation for improvement. *Quality Progress.* 1994;27(6):81–86.

4. Geller B, Craney JL, Bolhofner K, Nickelsburg MJ, Williams M, Zimerman B. Two-year prospective follow-up of children with a prepubertal and early adolescent bipolar disorder phenotype. *Am J Psychiatry.* 2002;159(6):927–933.

5. Chen Y, Kubzansky LD, VanderWeele TJ. Parental warmth and flourishing in mid-life. *Soc Sci Med.* 2019;220:65–72.

6. Petrill SA, Deater-Deckard K. Task orientation, parental warmth and SES account for a significant proportion of the shared environmental variance in general cognitive ability in early childhood: evidence from a twin study. *Dev Sci.* 2004;7(1):25–32.

7. Kam CM, Greenberg MT, Bierman KL, et al. Maternal depressive symptoms and child social preference during the early school years: mediation by maternal warmth and child emotion regulation. *J Abnorm Child Psychol.* 2011;39(3):365–377.

8. Girard LC, Doyle O, Tremblay RE. Maternal warmth and toddler development: support for transactional models in disadvantaged families. *Eur Child & Adolesc Psychiatry.* 2017;26(4):497–507.

# Index